50 WAYS
to Control
Migraines

Proven Relief for Adult, Adolescent, and Child Migraine Sufferers

Ceabert J. Griffith, N.D., P.A.-C.

Contemporary Books

Chicago   New York   San Francisco   Lisbon   London   Madrid   Mexico City
Milan   New Delhi   San Juan   Seoul   Singapore   Sydney   Toronto

To all my esteemed teachers, colleagues, students, and patients, who taught me everything I know about headaches in general and migraines in particular.

Library of Congress Cataloging-in-Publication Data

Griffith, Ceabert J.
     50 ways to control migraines : proven relief for adult, adolescent, and child migraine sufferers / Ceabert J. Griffith.
         p.   cm.
     Includes bibliographical references and index.
     ISBN 0-658-02157-5 (alk. paper)
     1. Migraine—Popular Works.   I. Title: Fifty ways to control migraines.   II. Title.

RC392 .G75 2002
616.8'57—dc21   2002023420

Contemporary Books

A Division of The **McGraw·Hill** Companies

2 3 4 5 6 7 8 9 0   DOC/DOC   1 0 9 8 7 6 5 4 3

ISBN 0-658-02157-5

McGraw-Hill books are available at special quantity discounts to use as premiums and sales promotions, or for use in corporate training programs. For more information, please write to the Director of Special Sales, Professional Publishing, McGraw-Hill, Two Penn Plaza, New York, NY 10121-2298. Or contact your local bookstore.

The purpose of this book is to educate. It is sold with the understanding that the author and publisher shall have neither liability nor responsibility for any injury caused or alleged to be caused directly or indirectly by the information contained in this book. While every effort has been made to ensure the book's accuracy, its contents should not be construed as medical advice. Each person's health needs are unique. To obtain recommendations appropriate to your particular situation, please consult a qualified health care provider.

This book is printed on acid-free paper.

Contents

Foreword

Over the past few decades, a large body of scientific findings has advanced our understanding of migraine headache: how and why it develops; who gets it; and the complex changes that characterize a typical episode. The discovery of many antimigraine drugs and medicinal herbs has given patients and their doctors an impressive list of pharmaceutical options with which to treat this enigmatic disease. In addition, clinicians have uncovered the efficacy of various lifestyle and mind/body strategies, such as proper nutrition, stress management, and biofeedback. No question, our current knowledge of migraine headache and how to get rid of it is light-years more advanced than even twenty years ago.

My good friend and associate, Dr. Bert Griffith, has carefully compiled these cutting-edge scientific findings and put them under one cover in the form of *50 Ways to Control Migraines*. Drawing on his background in both family and natural medicine, Dr. Griffith has prepared a well-written and easy-to-read book that will be well received. While this handbook is primarily written for migraine sufferers and their advocates, I'm sure that health care policy makers, health care administrators, health educators, and others will find this book an indispensable "go-to" reference.

As a family medicine physician, I found *50 Ways to Control Migraines* to be a comprehensive clinical primer on migraine headache. I plan to recommend it to my patients and to refer to it in my clinical practice. I am confident that primary care and specialty doctors, physician assistants, nurse practitioners, physical therapists, psychologists, optometrists, and other medical professionals will find this book similarly helpful. This book will empower you, as a migraineur, to become a proactive participant in the evaluation and management of your recurrent headache pain. Indeed, you'll be prepared to not only be your own advocate, but to help your health care provider help you reduce or eliminate your suffering. I agree with Dr. Griffith that this book will offer employers, coworkers, and friends and family of migraine sufferers invaluable insight into what the migraineur experiences and how best to help her or him.

I applaud your efforts to expand your fund of migraine knowledge, and wish you all the very best. Happy reading!

Keith Morita, M.D.
Chief of Medical Staff
USAF Hospital
Yokota Air Base, Japan

Acknowledgments

I'm deeply indebted to the dozens of people who lent uncon-
ditional support to this project. I apologize to those supporters
whose names I neglect to mention. Firstly, I'd like especially
to thank my editors, Kathryn Keil and Hudson Perigo, who
provided me with the coaching and encouragement needed to
give life to this work. Their passionate support of this project,
wise counsel, and firm deadline mandates provided the backdrop for my motivation and productivity.

No book is ever written without the unwavering support
of family, friends, mentors, and colleagues, and this book is
no exception. I owe my highest gratitude to my dear wife,
Yuko Kinjo Griffith, who has been my biggest fan over the
years and who cheerfully tolerated my frequent absences from
family gatherings during the time I spent researching and
writing this book. My four wonderful children—Michael,
Vanessa, Kevin, and Meg—provided the daily inspiration
needed to help me stay focused on my work. My parents,
Ceabert and Dora Griffith, and my late grandmother, Beryl
DaCosta, were my inspirations from the beginning.

With esteemed friends like Joel Paulino, M.D.; Marc Hawkins, P.A.-C.; John Harris, M.P.A.S., P.A.-C.; José Ramon DeClet, M.P.A.S., P.A.-C.; Jim Allen, M.P.A.S., P.A.-C.; and Dave Elger, M.A., offering timely suggestions, this book was destined to be a reality. With perennial mentors like Rod Hooker, P.A., Ph.D.; George L. White, Jr., P.A.-C., M.S.P.H., Ph.D.; and Steve Tiger, P.A.-C., providing invaluable counsel, I was bound to put out a masterful product. Finally, my sincere thanks to Mr. Steven Rowland and my other bosses and coworkers at U.S. Marine Corps Community Services, Okinawa, who created a perfectly stress-free work environment that left me with intact writing skills and creativity at the end of an arduous workday.

Ceabert J. Griffith, P.A.-C., N.D.

A Note on Terminology

At the back of the book you will find a comprehensive glossary of headache and associated terms. I suggest that you browse the glossary to familiarize yourself with the terminology before reading the book, and refer to the glossary thereafter as needed.

Throughout the book the terms *provider, clinician, health care practitioner,* and *health care provider* refer to health care professionals who practice medicine or support the practice of medicine in the United States, Canada, Britain, and elsewhere. These practitioners include allopathic physicians, physician assistants, and naturopathic doctors. Other health practitioners who evaluate and treat individuals with headache pain include nurse practitioners, chiropractors, psychologists, acupuncturists, optometrists, dietitians, occupational therapists, and pharmacists.

Introduction

As far as Joanne was concerned, only three things in life were certain: death, taxes, and her monthly headaches. Joanne had long accepted the first two inevitabilities but had vowed to get rid of the agonizing head pain that had virtually imprisoned her since the summer following her eleventh birthday. Despite her best efforts, Joanne's headaches had been unresponsive to maximum dosages of a variety of pain-killers, including extra-strength acetaminophen, naproxen, and ibuprofen. The accompanying nausea, diarrhea, mental confusion, irritability, and total weakness she experienced were downright disabling.

At the urging of her mother—herself a chronic headache sufferer—Joanne finally made it to see a family physician. The doctor recommended that Joanne keep a detailed diary of each headache episode, noting the date and time; location, intensity, and duration of the pain; associated symptoms; dietary intake; activities; and menstrual status. This strategy, reasoned the doctor, might reveal a pain pattern that showed, for example, a relationship between her headaches and something in her diet, and help to develop an effective treatment and prevention plan. The physician also prescribed an antimigraine medication, a balanced diet, and an aerobic exercise program, and asked Joanne to return for a follow-up visit in three months.

Joanne returned to her doctor feeling liberated and filled with optimism. With the help of three months of meticulous headache diary entries, Joanne's doctor was able to determine that she was experiencing menstrual migraine. The doctor continued Joanne on her diet and an antimigraine drug that was to be taken before the onset of and during her menstrual period. He also recommended she continue keeping a headache diary to help gauge the efficacy of her medication and diet. Finally, he suggested that Joanne buy a good book on migraine headache to educate and empower herself about this very complex and enigmatic condition.

Within six months, Joanne was completely headache free, getting only an occasional nonmigraine-type headache. She no longer misses work or social events and doesn't distance herself from friends and loved ones. Her employer, coworkers, and friends no longer regard her as weird and unreliable. Nearly two decades after her headaches began, Joanne is finally in control of her life and ready to lift herself out of a world of despair, anger, anxiety, depression, and loneliness.

Sadly, Joanne's headache story is far from unique. Each day, an estimated twenty million people in the United States experience some form of head pain. Worldwide, an estimated 93 percent of all men and 99 percent of all women will experience one or more headache episodes during their lifetimes, making headache the most prevalent of all human diseases![1] Migraine headache—the second most prevalent type of headache behind tension-type headache—affects between twenty-five and thirty million American adults and about one million children.[2]

Chronic headache—the biggest reason for disability payments to American workers—is also expensive to evaluate and treat. Indeed, forty-five million people in the United States seek medical care for headaches each year. The National Headache Foundation estimates that businesses lose about $50 billion annually to absenteeism and payment of medical benefits to headache sufferers.[3] Migraines alone cost employers and patients an astounding $11 billion a year.[4]

Is headache a relatively recent disease that came into its own during the last century? As it turns out, it's not. Indeed, historical accounts show that headache has been around about as long as mankind has. In fact, the modern name *migraine* is not so modern; it's derived from the term *hemikrania,* meaning "half a head," used by second-century Greek physician and writer Galen to describe the classic one-sided head pain that his migraine sufferers experienced. Many recorded accounts from ancient civilizations stretching from Egypt to Sumeria and India tell vivid stories of headache sufferers who were virtually consumed by their disease.

Although our prehistoric and premodern ancestors suffered from the scourge of chronic headache, we don't have to do so. The good news is that recent headache research has discovered significant evidence pointing to the causes of migraines. These findings have led to great improvements in the approach to the management of migraine headache, including drug and nondrug therapy. Despite these advances, however, the cornerstone of migraine management remains self-care with physician guidance. As a migraine sufferer—or the parent, spouse, relative, or friend of one — you need to know that headache self-care begins with a thorough education about the condition: what it is, what it isn't, what causes it, and how to manage it.

My objective in writing this book is to help to bridge the communication gap between health care providers and migraine patients. Recent surveys of patients with chronic illnesses (such as heart disease, cancer, and migraines) show that doctors and other health care professionals don't spend enough time educating their patients. This growing "disconnection" results from time constraints imposed by the way most Americans get health care. Managed-care networks place greater emphasis on seeing larger numbers of patients in fewer contact hours. This leaves health care professionals with less time to effectively educate their patients. As a result, individuals who want to understand the nature of their disease must seize the initiative if they are to tap into alternative resources. As a holistic doctor, I believe that information management — via patient education books like this one — is the best way to close the doctor-patient information gap.

Reading *50 Ways to Control Migraines* will arm you with the migraine headache education needed to regain control of your life. But I'd like to emphasize caution. No health care education book — no matter how well researched — can be a substitute for a medical doctor or other qualified health care professional. Your physician and other medical providers are best qualified to evaluate and prescribe the most effective management for your migraines. It is my hope that you, your family and friends, your employer, and your health care practitioners will read this book, use it, and recommend it as a single-source guide to halt, or reduce, the frequency, intensity, and duration of your migraine episodes.

PART ONE

Understanding Migraine Headaches

1. Learn the Basics About Pain

What would a totally pain-free life be like? To begin with, it would mean no more migraine headache! In addition, it would mean that we would not flinch if we broke a finger during an accident, and surgeons could remove diseased appendixes without subjecting the patient to the risk of general anesthesia. Moreover, there would be no pain to go along with the incessant bleeding from a large gash in our leg. But is *not* being able to feel pain good for us?

Pain has one crucial function: to warn us that something harmful has occurred in the body. Pain warns us of dangers that, if ignored, can lead to physical harm or even death. For example, unknowingly touching a hot curling iron without the ability to sense that your hand is burning would lead to complete destruction of your skin, muscles, tendons, ligaments, bones—indeed, your entire hand. Do this a couple of times and you'll destroy your entire body. As you can see, pain serves an important life-preserving function.

What makes you feel pain and how does it all happen? According to well-known headache specialists Drs. Alan Rapoport and Fred Sheftell, pain complements the interaction between the nerves that monitor your environment and your brain.[1] Your ability to feel pain is made possible by two bodily systems: the endocrine system, which contains the glands and hormones that help the glands communicate with each other; and the nervous system, comprising the brain and forty-five miles of spinal and peripheral nerves. The perception of pain is very complicated, but very fast. When you are hit on the arm by the ball during a softball game, for instance, the nerve endings in your skin below the point of impact get stimulated (irritated) and send a message to the brain. A series of chemicals called *neurotransmitters* help speed the transmission of the message. After receiving the message, the brain interprets it as pain and dispatches a response message directing you to withdraw your arm, ice it, or otherwise protect it.

How you respond to being hit during a football game — ignore the pain and keep playing or stop and writhe in agony — is individualized and determines how you perceive and respond to other forms of pain. Perhaps based on life experiences and expectations, each person develops his or her own *pain threshold,* the weakest stimulus that a person perceives and interprets as pain. *Pain tolerance* refers to the degree of severity a person assigns to a pain stimulus. Thus, the severity of pain is somewhat subjective and mostly relative. This is why one person exhibits a dramatic response to a splinter in her finger, while another easily shakes off the contusion caused by a sixty-pound steel ball falling on his foot.

An individual's pain threshold can be lowered by a number of psychological factors, such as emotional stress and depression, which affect the secretion of neurotransmitters like serotonin (discussed later). Some pain researchers believe that some forms of headache pain are related to how an individual perceives and responds to external stimuli, such as rush hour traffic or conflict with a coworker. The stress of slow-moving traffic may cause some persons to clench their teeth ("Why do so many people have to choose the same highway as me?") and develop a migraine flare. Others respond with complete calm ("I can't do anything about this traffic; besides, this is the only way to get to work") and never develop headache.

2. Know Why Your Head Aches

Hippocrates, the renowned fifth-century B.C. Greek physician, was the first to propose a biological model for headache pain. His contemporaries were skeptical; instead of looking at headache as a symptom of a disease, they regarded headache pain as the work of demons. After the Dark Ages, scientists—many of them headache sufferers—began to realize that there was more to headaches than demons, and started publishing a number of rudimentary, biologically based hypotheses.

However, it wasn't until 1940 that Harold Wolff and John Graham found that the drug ergotamine, still used today to treat migraine headache, narrowed blood vessels and brought relief to migraineurs and other headache sufferers. Further biological phenomena of migraine and other types of headaches have since been discovered and elucidated. Headache clinicians and researchers are now more knowledgeable about the very complicated anomalies involved in the development of migraines and other forms of headaches.

A most significant scientific finding in the past three decades is that, for the most part, headache results from abnormal biological mechanisms. For example, most primary headache sufferers (people whose headaches have no identifiable cause) may have an inborn predisposition for their headaches. However, not everyone biologically predisposed to migraines and other primary headaches gets them. Apparently, the inherited propensity must be triggered by external factors, such as air pollution and bright lights, or internal factors, such as depression and low blood sugar. As headache scientist Dr. Michel Ferrari of Leiden University in the Netherlands said, "Certain patients will have a genetic predisposition but will develop migraine only when other, presumably environmental, factors are involved."[2]

In addition to the hereditary tendency for migraines and other headaches, researchers found an environmental aspect to chronic headache. Some clinicians and headache researchers feel that the development of headache can be a learned behavior, where biologically predisposed children develop headaches by observing parents, siblings, or relatives during headache flare-ups.[3]

There is also a distinct physiological aspect of headache pain. Although it sounds like science fiction, the human brain itself can't feel pain. This means that if a neurosurgeon cuts into the brain tissue of an awake patient during brain surgery, the patient will not feel pain! This has to do with the fact that the brain lacks the network of nerves that transmit pain messages. The pain a patient undergoing brain surgery feels originates in the nerves that innervate the blood vessels (the tubelike plumbing that transports blood) and muscles on the scalp, face, and neck. The nerves outside the brain sense the prick of a pin and send the sensory input (message) to the brain, which interprets the sensation as pain. Headache results when these pain-sensitive structures outside the brain are stimulated, usually by pressure from surrounding tissues.

Headache pain is therefore a symptom that indicates an abnormality in a system of the body, much like discharge from the ear is a symptom that a germ has invaded the ear canal. One of the foremost scientific discoveries in the 1960s and 1970s was the role of the brain chemical serotonin (sometimes referred to by its chemical name 5-HT) in the development of headache. Researchers have shown that, for reasons still unknown, serotonin covers the blood vessels of the brain, causing them to narrow.[4] This in turn leads to a drop in blood serotonin levels, expansion (widening) of the blood vessels, and the throbbing pain of a migraine flare-up. Other brain chemicals involved in the development of headache include substance P, bradykinin, dopamine, and norepinephrine.

Headaches are also linked to hormonal factors. Scientists at the University of Mississippi Medical Center demonstrated that women who experience changes in their gynecological health, such as the development of ovarian cysts and irregular menstrual cycles, are twice as likely to develop chronic headaches as are women without such changes.

3. Know the Major Classifications of Headaches

Because there are numerous types of headaches, each presenting with its own set of symptoms, a standard system of identifying each type is necessary. To enhance treatment efficacy and facilitate follow-up, it's important to identify the type of headache you have. For example, a menstrual migraine headache is managed differently from a tension-type headache.

Prior to 1988, there were no standard definitions for the many kinds of headaches. The International Headache Society (IHS), an organization of the world's foremost headache scientists and clinicians, has identified 129 types of head and neck pain affecting humans, and has published the definitions and diagnostic criteria of all headache disorders. The IHS divides all headaches into two major categories: (1) *primary headaches* and (2) *secondary headaches.*[5] Primary headaches, which include cluster and migraine headaches and make up 95 percent of all headaches, are not caused by any specific medical problem. Although frustrating and downright depressing, rarely are primary headaches a cause for concern.

Conversely, secondary or organic headaches are those that result from an identifiable medical problem, as listed below. Secondary headaches, which can be either benign or life threatening, cause less than 5 percent of all headaches.

IHS also classifies headaches as either acute or chronic. An acute headache is a single episode, typically of short duration, and not related to previous, recurrent episodes. The acute headache sufferer will have a full and complete recovery without lasting effects. Chronic headaches, such as those caused by migraine, represent a distinct pattern of head pain that recurs for many months and even years with varying frequency and duration.

Non–Life-Threatening Causes of Headaches

- Allergies
- Sinus problems
- High blood pressure
- Vision problems
- Temporomandibular joint (TMJ) syndrome
- Trauma
- Hormonal imbalance
- Temporal arteritis
- Pseudotumor cerebri
- Cervicogenic headache
- Drugs such as painkillers, antibiotics, and high blood pressure pills
- Dehydration
- Alcohol overindulgence
- Spinal tap
- Physical exertion
- Carbon monoxide poisoning
- Fever
- Emotional stress

Life-Threatening Causes of Headaches

- Brain tumor
- Meningitis
- Encephalitis
- Ruptured aneurysm
- Stroke

4. Learn Who Gets Chronic Headaches

Chronic headache affects everyone; it knows no racial, ethnic, cultural, gender, or geographic boundaries. Therefore, Japanese Americans, American Indians, and Caucasians all suffer chronic headache. Men, women, adolescents, middle-aged individuals, and the elderly are all potential victims.

Even the youngest among us can be chronic headache sufferers. Dr. Irving Fish, director of pediatric neurology at New York University Medical Center in New York City, said in an interview with CNN on June 25, 1999, "About 85 percent of children by the time they're seventeen have had headaches severe enough to mention them to their physicians."

Chronic headache is a worldwide affliction. Approximately 59 percent of adult Canadians report some form of acute or chronic headache. The Migraine Association of Canada reports that 3.2 million Canadians suffer from migraine headache (The Migraine Association of Canada: http://www.migraine.ca/STROKE.HTM). The American People's Medical Society estimates that 11 percent of the U.S. population suffers from migraine headache.[6] Zimbabwe public health officials estimate that 20 percent of the population suffers from chronic headache, while in New Zealand the number stands at 49 percent. In the United States, Britain, and Canada, more women than men suffer from chronic headache, including migraines.

5. Recognize the Social and Economic Impact of Headaches

Chronic headache is a debilitating disorder that can negatively impact the quality of life of adults, children, and adolescents; workplace productivity; and social relationships, and can induce emotional scars. The National Headache Foundation estimates that untold billions of dollars are spent annually in the United States on the care of head pain—$11 billion in health care costs to treat migraines alone, and $4 billion on over-the-counter painkillers.[7] Employers may pay as much as five thousand dollars a year in health premiums for employed headache sufferers.

6. Study the Historical Perspectives on Headaches

Ancient, medieval, and modern history is full of accounts of headache suffering. Many famous religious, political, cultural, academic, and military leaders and other contributors to civilization were or are known chronic headache sufferers.

In the New Testament, Saul of Tarsus suffered from recurrent visual disturbances, piercing head pain, and stomach upset, symptoms reminiscent of migraine headache. The *Atharvaveda* of India, a book about magic formulas that was penned between 1500 and 800 B.C., contains essays about headache. Early Greek history is also replete with accounts of headache suffering. One tablet at Epidaurus (circa 1250 B.C.) described Agestratos's recurrent headaches.[8] Hippocrates (circa 460–370 B.C.) accurately chronicled the symptoms of a male patient suffering from what is now known to be migraine headache:

> Most of the time he seemed to see something shining before him like a light, usually in part of the right eye; at the end of a moment, a violent pain supervened in the right temple, then in all the head and neck, where the head is attached to the spine . . . vomiting, when it became possible, was able to divert the pain and render it more moderate.[9]

Skulls bearing evidence of holes cut into them to treat headache (a practice referred to as trepanning) have been discovered in Europe and South America.[10] The Incas of ancient Peru used trepanning to treat chronic headache pain. South Pacific islanders used it to treat epilepsy, insanity, and recurrent headache as recently as the seventeenth century.[11] I can't imagine too many people surviving the ordeal of such a drastic treatment. Thank goodness, trepanning has since been supplanted by modern—and less painful—measures to manage headache pain.

Fast forwarding to modern times, known chronic headache sufferers include English naturalist Charles Darwin, English dramatist George Bernard Shaw, psychoanalyst Sigmund Freud, and political economist Karl Marx. In the United States, third president Thomas Jefferson, Civil War general and eighteenth U.S. president Ulysses S. Grant, and inventor Alexander Graham Bell were all known to suffer chronic bouts of head pain. In more recent times, chronic headache sufferers include Hall of Fame basketball player Kareem Abdul-Jabbar and the king of rock 'n roll, the late Elvis Presley.

Fortunately for us, these brave headache sufferers didn't give in to their recurrent head pain; in spite of their chronic suffering, they went on to become giants in their respective professional fields. They became major influences in shaping our culture. Indeed, when it comes to headache suffering, history is on your side. Migraine headaches can be effectively conquered!

7. Don't Fall for Chronic Headache Myths

"Not tonight, honey, I have a headache." This statement has become common vernacular in popular sitcoms and movies. As innocent as this line might seem, it has served to desensitize the general public about the true nature of headache pain and the plight of chronic headache sufferers. Indeed, society has come to view headache as an insignificant medical problem, probably because head pain cannot be seen or measured like blood pressure or cholesterol. The prevailing assumption is that the chronic sufferer is not really sick; she just isn't capable of intimacy, and uses headache as the perfect excuse.

These negative stereotypical portrayals of headache and its chronic sufferers spawn many myths about the nature of the condition and the psychology and motivation of headache sufferers. Eventually, people who don't suffer chronic headaches come to regard the chronic headache sufferer as pretentious, whose aims are to get sympathy and deceive family, friends, coworkers, employers, insurance companies, and society at large.

8. Focus on Migraine Facts

MYTH: Migraine headache is not a real medical problem like high blood pressure or kidney failure.
FACT: Many world-renowned headache researchers and clinicians, such as Dr. Richard Lipton of Albert Einstein College of Medicine in the Bronx, New York, and Dr. Seymour Solomon of the American Council on Headache Education, have shown that migraine headache is a legitimate *biological* disorder.

MYTH: Migraine sufferers have hypersensitivity to pain. People with migraines are just abnormally aware of every little change in their bodies.
FACT: People who dismiss migraines as "just a headache" undoubtedly have never experienced the throbbing, debilitating head pain of migraine that makes it difficult to concentrate at work or school, socialize, or enjoy a close relationship

with family and friends. There is no question that the degree of sensitivity to pain can vary from person to person, but there is no scientific evidence that migraineurs are more sensitive to pain sensation than their nonheadache peers.

MYTH: Migraine sufferers have poor coping skills. People with migraines don't know how to adequately deal with fear, sadness, anger, and other emotions.
FACT: Centuries of clinical experience and years of sound scientific research have conclusively shown that migraine headache is heralded by a number of complicated biochemical and physical changes in the brain. There is no doubt that psychological factors such as stress, anger, and other emotions can *trigger* migraine headaches, but in the majority of cases the biological propensity must be in place. Indeed, many persons who get stressed out and angry do not experience migraine headaches, while large numbers of headache sufferers get head pain without getting angry or stressed out.

MYTH: Migraine headache results from having a type A personality: "If you were not so darn competitive, ambitious, goal oriented, and impatient you wouldn't be cursed with those chronic headaches."
FACT: The scientific literature unequivocally doesn't support the theory of a "migraine personality."[12] In fact, many people who fit the "migraine personality" profile don't suffer from migraines; and many people with migraine headaches are not competitive, goal oriented, and impatient. This myth just doesn't hold water when held up to scientific scrutiny!

MYTH: Migraine headache is a woman's disease—that's why many more women than men get them.

FACT: Most women do not get migraine headaches and a fair share of men suffer from them (more than 30 percent of sufferers are men), which hardly makes migraine a gender-specific condition. Women who suffer from migraines clearly have hormonal factors that influence their head pain. The fact is, men, too, experience hormonally based chronic headaches. Cluster headaches, which affect six times more men than women, are felt to be related to the male hormone testosterone, similar to estrogen's role in the development of migraines.

MYTH: Smart and rich people don't get migraines; only uneducated and economically disadvantaged folks get them.

FACT: There is no question that migraine headache is an equal opportunity offender, affecting persons at all levels of socioeconomic and intellectual endowment. As mentioned previously, Charles Darwin and Thomas Jefferson—arguably two of the most intellectually gifted statesmen in the past few hundred years—suffered from recurrent headaches that were more than likely migraines. Both Elizabeth Taylor and Whoopi Goldberg are rich and famous, and they suffer from chronic headaches. In other words, chronic headaches, including migraines, can happen to anyone.

MYTH: "Migraine is all in your head; ignore the pain and it will eventually go away."

FACT: No question, migraine headache *is* in the head. But it isn't *all* in the head. Migraine pain is as real as the pain of angina or a broken leg. Even though scientists haven't discovered all the pieces to the migraine puzzle, recent breakthrough findings clearly show the complicated biological processes involved in migraines. Some people predisposed to migraine head pain also have to contend with the issue of foods, the environment, and other factors that can trigger their headaches.

9. Identify Migraine Triggers

Identifying headache triggers can go a long way in helping you control or get rid of your headaches. Some forms of migraines are triggered by environmental factors (e.g., bright or flickering lights), foods (e.g., caffeine), everyday medicines (e.g., ibuprofen), and social habits (e.g., smoking).[13] Next to stress, dietary triggers play a larger role in headache activation than any other factor.

Factors that trigger migraines are not the biological *causes* of headaches; instead, these factors *activate* or trigger headaches when predisposed migraineurs are exposed to them. The exact mechanisms by which headache triggers precipitate a migraine attack remain a mystery to scientists. However, many experts speculate that the offending trigger causes an irregular pattern of electrical activity in the outer layer of the brain called the cortex.[14]

Headache triggers aren't universal; different people are affected by different triggers, and many migraine sufferers are not bothered by any triggers. The best way to determine if you are a victim of headache triggers, and what they are, is to keep a headache diary to see if your attacks coincide with a particular trigger. Refer to the following lists of headache triggers to help you fill out your headache diary.

High Altitude and Air Travel

The sudden changes in oxygen pressure that occur with air travel cause the blood vessels in the scalp, which are hypersensitive to changes in the pressure of oxygen, to swell, setting off a migraine attack. A drop in oxygen pressure also reduces the amount of oxygen going to the brain. Indeed, some migraineurs report headache flares during airplane travel, when ascending mountains and large hills, or during scuba diving. Predisposed migraineurs who live at elevations over 6,000 feet or who drive up or down steep inclines also report episodic flare-ups of their head pain.

Migraineurs who experience attacks during changes in altitude should consider having extra oxygen available during air travel. If you decide to climb a mountain or large hill, do so only after you've become physically fit. Gradually ascend in stages, allowing time for acclimatization, when possible. When traveling across time zones, especially west-to-east travel, be cognizant of the potential for headache flares associated with a time-zone switch and jet lag.

Don't forget to continually hydrate yourself, preferably with water, to guard against dehydration caused by sweating or the dry air inside an airplane. When flying, bring your own water and avoid alcoholic beverages. Physicians often prescribe the drug Diamox or corticosteroids for altitude sickness. Vitamin C, which promotes the circulation of oxygen throughout the body, may also help to reduce the negative effects of high altitude.

Weather Changes

Changes in weather patterns can cause changes in the body's internal environment, triggering migraine in sensitive individuals. Some migraine sufferers report headache flare-ups when there's a change in outside temperature, humidity level, and barometric pressure. Others report frequent attacks during the first few weeks of spring and autumn. Still others are affected by so-called "ill winds," such as the southern California Santa Ana, the hot, dry winds of the Arizona desert, the Argentine zonda, the Israeli sharav, and the Balkan bora.

Symptoms of weather-induced migraines include fatigue, poor concentration, anxiety, and lethargy. If your migraines are touched off by changes in the weather, be sure to have a well thought out plan for sudden changes in barometric pressure. Ask your health care practitioner if you are a candidate for prophylactic headache medicines.

Air Pollution

Many migraineurs trace their head pain to exposure to heavy smog, vehicle exhaust fumes, industrial smoke, and other air pollutants. Their headaches stop upon leaving the offending environment. Medical scientists believe the problem is partly caused by high levels of carbon monoxide competing with oxygen for space on the oxygen-carrying pigments in the blood.

Besides relocating, the best way to combat air pollutants is to limit outside activities on days when air pollution is high. Because asthmatics and others with health problems are affected by air pollution, most TV and radio stations and Internet news organizations routinely alert listeners and viewers on days when air pollution is expected to reach unhealthy levels. If you take annual vacations, try to plan your time away during peak pollution days. Again, most news organizations keep historical records of air pollution patterns and make this information available to the general public.

Other Environmental Factors

Loud music, high-frequency machinery, airplanes flying overhead, and other sources of loud noise can cause migraine attacks. The best way to combat loud noise is avoidance, but when this is not possible, you should use earplugs. Some migraine sufferers promptly experience headaches on exposure to strong odors such as colognes and perfumes, tobacco smoke, petroleum products, and room deodorizers.[17] Again, avoidance is the best way to deal with these triggers.

11. Avoid Dietary Migraine Triggers

The precise mechanisms by which foodstuffs trigger headaches remain unclear. The most common dietary migraine triggers are chocolate, monosodium glutamate (MSG), amines, nitrates, sulfites, artificial sweeteners, and nuts. Gamma-aminobutyric acid (GABA), salt, ice cream, onions, beans, caffeine, and citrus fruits are also common triggers.

Chocolate

Chocolate contains a number of substances, including theobromides, the amine phenylethylamine, and ground cacao, that have been shown to trigger migraine headaches in some sufferers. Phenylethylamine can affect the blood vessel tone, triggering migraine and migrainelike headaches. Keep in mind that plain and bitter chocolate contain higher levels of phenylethylamine than milk chocolate and white chocolate.

Some migraineurs crave chocolate just before a migraine attack. Interestingly, while some migraineurs report that chocolate triggers a migraine attack, others find that chocolate actually *stops* their headaches.[18] While chocolate might be very appealing to the taste and psyche, if it brings on a migraine you'll have to stop eating it. If you have to have a chocolate-like substance in your diet, you can switch to carob, a type of naturally sweet, ground-up bean pod with the same consistency as chocolate.[19] Carob can be purchased as bars that look similar to chocolate bars. There are even dairy-free carob bars for those who are lactose intolerant. Other chocolate substitutes include penuche and toffee.

Monosodium Glutamate

Monosodium glutamate (MSG), a derivative of the amino acid glutamic acid, is a food flavor enhancer found in many food additives and in most packaged, canned, and frozen entrées. Chemically similar to gamma-aminobutyric acid (see page 25), MSG is also used to enhance the flavor of commercial soups, gravies, hot dogs, and many other foods.

The U.S. Department of Agriculture mandates that all labels of processed meat and poultry products list MSG and other food additives by name to alert people who are hypersensitive to these enhancers. Other names for MSG include "hydrolyzed vegetable protein," "textured vegetable protein," "flavoring," "hydrolyzed plant protein," and "natural flavor." MSG is a common food enhancer in foods prepared in Chinese restaurants. For example, a seven-ounce bowl of wonton soup contains about three grams of MSG, a sufficient amount to cause a migraine flare-up in a predisposed individual.[20]

MSG–associated headache usually starts less than thirty minutes after consuming the additive. The headache commonly feels like a bandlike pressure around the forehead and pressure or throbbing over the temples. Other symptoms include dizziness, pressure in the chest, and abdominal cramps. The best treatment for MSG–induced headache is avoidance. Get into the habit of reading food labels.

Amines

Some migraineurs report attacks after ingesting foods containing amines, a group of vasoactive, nitrogen-based protein components.[21] These substances cause the blood vessels to narrow and then expand, touching off a headache. The following amines have been implicated:

- Dopamine in legumes, such as peanuts, peas, broad beans, and soy.

- Tyramine in aged foods, such as cheese, yogurt, buttermilk, sourdough, and overripe bananas. Red wine, beer, dried or pickled meat, salami, nuts, figs, raisins, avocados, and fish also contain high amounts of tyramine.

- Histamine in cold-water fish, such as salmon and tuna.

- Phenylethylamine in chocolate.

- Octopamine and synephrine in citrus fruits.

- Tryptamine in tomatoes and pineapples.

Onions

Some migraineurs report that onions trigger their headaches. Onions contain tyramine, which can cause migraine flares in susceptible individuals. See the discussion on tyramine under Amines.

Beans

Beans contain dopamine, which can trigger headaches in susceptible migraineurs by affecting blood vessel tone. See the discussion on dopamine under Amines.

Nitrites and Nitrates

Nitrites and nitrates are a group of chemicals that are used as preservatives in many canned foods. These substances — referred to as sodium nitrite, potassium nitrite, and nitric acid — are added to foods to prevent botulism, an often-fatal form of food poisoning. Additionally, nitrates and nitrites give foods their pink or reddish color and distinctly "cured" taste. Bacon, salami, hot dogs, bologna, and sausage contain these chemicals. In fact, the nitrite in hot dogs is the cause of what some clinicians still call "hot-dog headaches."

Nitrates and nitrites trigger migraine headaches by expanding (dilating) blood vessels in the head and neck. These substances act on blood vessels in a similar manner to nitroglycerine used to treat angina. Indeed, a common side effect of using nitroglycerine is an agonizing, migraine-like head pain.

Sulfites

Sulfites refer to a group of chemicals used as preservatives in foods, alcohol, and drugs. These chemicals give fruits and vegetables a "fresh" appearance and, despite their ban, are still used by some restaurants to enhance the appearance of salads. Wine makers also add sulfites to their products to inhibit bacterial growth in wine. Chemical names for sulfites include potassium bisulfite, sodium sulfite, and sulfur dioxide.

Sulfites can be found in foods such as soups, sauces, gravy mixes, frozen potato products, dried fruits, and avocado dip. Beer and wine also contain "sulfiting" agents. Drugs that contain sulfites include intravenous and spray preparations.

Sulfite sensitivity causes symptoms such as flushing, difficulty breathing, nausea, vomiting, hives, and headache. Extreme cases of sulfite sensitivity have led to loss of consciousness and death.

Artificial Sweeteners

Aspartame, the artificial sweetener sold as Equal, Spoonful, and Nutrasweet, has been implicated as a headache trigger in susceptible migraineurs.[22] This sweetener is an almost odorless crystalline powder with an intensely sweet taste, and is derived from aspartic acid and the metyl ester of phenylalanine. It is found in many everyday products such as soft drinks, puddings, yogurt, chewing gum, and some desserts. If your migraine is triggered by these food products, be sure to avoid aspartame-containing foods and drinks.

Nuts

Tree nut and peanut sensitivity affects over three million Americans and has been known to touch off migraines. Peanuts contain large amounts of dopamine, a vasoactive substance known to act on the blood vessels in the head and neck. Walnuts, pecans, almonds, coconut, cashews, and pistachios can also trigger migraines in sensitive individuals.

Gamma-Aminobutyric Acid

Gamma-aminobutyric acid (GABA), found in the human brain, kidneys, heart, and lungs, and naturally in some plants, is a chemical that helps transmit messages between nerve cells. Chemically similar to MSG, GABA consumption has been implicated by some migraine sufferers as a head-pain trigger. Doctors use GABA to treat epilepsy and high blood pressure.

Salt

Salt or sodium may play a role in triggering migraines in some individuals. Sodium is believed to cause platelets to clump together, a condition that leads to vascular headaches. Sodium is found in high concentration in many canned foods and food additives. Two ounces of Parmesan cheese, for example, contain 1,056 milligrams of sodium. Your daily intake of salt should not exceed 2,400 milligrams.

Ice Cream

Some migraine sufferers experience pain behind the eyes, deep behind the bridge of the nose, or in the temples when they eat ice cream or other very cold foods. Ice-cream–induced headache pain usually lasts about twenty to thirty seconds. The exact mechanism by which ice cream sets off headaches in these individuals is not known, but some plausible theories have been published. Headache specialists Drs. Alan Rapoport and Fred Sheftell believe that the impact of the cold of the ice cream on the warm tissues of the roof of the mouth and throat induces nerve and blood vessel changes that lead to the characteristic head pain.

If you suffer from ice cream headaches, you can avoid them by eating smaller bites and warming up the ice cream slightly in the front of your mouth before it hits your throat.[23] Between bites, hold the ice cream in front of your mouth for a few seconds until the roof of your mouth and throat cool slightly.

Caffeine

Found in many foods, drinks, and medications, caffeine has been implicated as a common migraine trigger. Research shows that excessive usage, as well as the sudden stoppage of caffeine intake, can trigger various headaches. Like nicotine, excessive caffeine narrows blood vessels excessively, lowering blood flow to the brain and setting off vascular headaches.

If your headaches are affected by caffeine, you should not take in more than 300 to 400 milligrams of caffeine—the amount in four cups of brewed coffee or five cans of cola-containing sodas—per day. Table 1 lists the caffeine content of some common caffeinated drinks, foods, and drugs.

Table 1

Caffeine in Some Common Drinks, Foods, and Medicines

Source	Estimated caffeine (in milligrams)
Brewed coffee, one cup (five ounces)	100–150
Instant coffee, one cup	85–100
Decaffeinated coffee, one cup	2–4
Cocoa, one cup	40–55
Chocolate bar	25
Cola	40–60
Anacin	32
Bromo-Seltzer	32
Cope	32
Darvon Compound	32
Excedrin	65
Midol	32
Pre-mens	30
Vanquish	33

Reducing caffeine intake can lead to rebound dilation of blood vessels, and this can trigger withdrawal headaches. The typical caffeine-withdrawal headache sufferer drinks lots of coffee at work and little or none on his or her days off, and develops throbbing headaches while away from work. If this describes you and you are trying to stop using caffeine, you should gradually reduce your intake over a three- to seven-day period. Check with your doctor for more advice on how to reduce or stop your caffeine consumption.

Fruits

Citrus fruits, which contain octopamine and synephrine, can cause headache flare-ups in predisposed migraineurs. The most commonly implicated fruits are oranges, grape-fruits, lemons, and limes. Overripe bananas, which contain high levels of tyramine, can also trigger headaches in some people. Most dried fruit, which contains high levels of sulfites (see page 24), can also cause migraine attacks. Unsulfited dried fruit is available at natural food stores.

12. Avoid Nutritional Deficiencies That Can Trigger Migraines

The unfortunate reality of the twenty-first century is that many of the foods we now consume contain more chemicals, pesticides, herbicides, and preservatives and fewer vitamins and minerals than even twenty years ago. A diet deficient in certain vitamins and minerals can activate migraines. Additionally, hypoglycemia (low blood sugar) can lead to migraine attacks.

Vitamin/Mineral Deficiency

Scientific studies have shown that a deficiency of certain vitamins and minerals can trigger migraines and other types of headaches. Other studies have shown that low levels of vitamins may also be related to recurrent headaches. Headaches also occur in people with chromium, copper, and iron deficiencies.[24]

In a 1991 study, adults with a history of both migraine and tension-type headaches were found to have significantly lower levels of magnesium compared to age-matched peers.[25] This important mineral has multiple bodily functions, such as to help stabilize the size of blood vessels, alter the function of serotonin, and prevent platelets from sticking together and thickening the blood. Magnesium deficiency leads to vasoconstriction and inflammation of the nerve endings that supply blood to the head and neck region, thereby triggering a migraine attack. Although studies looking at magnesium supplementation to prevent migraines have shown mixed results, migraineurs may find some relief by taking 300 to 400 milligrams of magnesium each day.[26] Good food sources of magnesium include green vegetables, nuts, and legumes.

Headache specialists Drs. Alan Rapoport and Fred Sheftell recommend multivitamins for persons whose diets lack some or all of the crucial vitamins.[27] However, megadoses of some vitamins—especially the fat-soluble vitamins, A, D, E, and K—may be bad for you. Fat-soluble vitamins can build up to life-threatening levels in fat cells. For example, high levels of vitamin A can induce pseudotumor cerebri, a condition characterized by a buildup of pressure in the brain. Check with your doctor before starting to take megadoses of any vitamins or minerals.

Hypoglycemia

Low blood sugar or hypoglycemia, caused by excessive dieting, prolonged fasting, or having too much insulin in the bloodstream, can set off migraines.[28] Insulin-dependent diabetics (people with abnormally high blood sugar) who take more insulin than they need are at risk of developing hypoglycemia (the opposite of diabetes).

Some migraineurs get a "hunger headache" if they forget to eat. The headache goes away after eating. Hypoglycemia induces hunger headaches by depriving the brain of glucose, the only substance the brain is able to use for energy. Hypoglycemia causes secretion of adrenaline, which, like amines (see page 23), is vasoactive; that is, it causes the blood vessels to narrow and then expand, activating a headache in susceptible migraineurs. This phenomenon is more likely to occur during the premenstrual period in women predisposed to menstrual migraine.

Symptoms of low blood sugar include anxiety, dizziness, mental confusion, feeling jittery, sweating, and clumsiness after missing a meal. To prevent a drop in blood sugar, eat frequent, small meals (approximately every three to four hours). Eat complex carbohydrates (e.g., whole grains and whole beans) and protein instead of foods made from refined sugar (e.g., donuts and most pastries). To maintain a normal blood sugar level during the night, some people may need to eat a light snack (e.g., crackers and cheese) before going to bed.

13. Refrain from Lifestyle Factors That Can Trigger Migraines

Emotional states, such as anxiety, stress, and depression, and lifestyle factors, such as changes in sleep pattern, have been blamed for triggering headaches in some individuals.

Stress and Other Emotional Factors

Although they can't be measured like the cholesterol level in your blood, the effects of emotional stress on our health are very significant. Many migraineurs trace the activation of their head pain to events that lead to excessive emotional stress. In fact, stress is one of the most common migraine triggers.[29] Factors connected to emotional stress include mental fatigue, anxiety, boredom, frustration, excessive worry, a poorly balanced diet, and depression.

Stress can cause physical and biochemical reactions in the body—the so-called "fight or flight" response—that mobilize the body to confront or flee from danger. During the fight or flight response the body releases a number of chemicals, including adrenaline and cortisol, that lead to the blood vessel changes that set off headache symptoms.

Like stress, anxiety, frustration, and anger can cause the body to secrete adrenaline that can narrow blood vessels and precipitate a migraine flare-up. Depression has been shown to increase the frequency and severity of migraine attacks in many migraineurs. This is not surprising since the chemical changes that occur with depression impair the body's ability to utilize the neurotransmitter serotonin. In the discussion of antidepressant drugs such as fluoxetine (Prozac) (see page 125), it will be clearer why depression can trigger migraines, and why antidepressant drugs work well to reduce the frequency and severity of migraine headaches in some people who suffer frequent migraine attacks.

Disrupted Sleep Pattern

The human brain is controlled by a biological clock that is inextricably connected to our food intake, emotional stress levels, and the sleep-wake cycle.[30] Any deviation from one's normal sleep pattern—either too much or too little sleep—can affect brain wave patterns and trigger headaches in some people. Be aware that a full night's sleep doesn't necessarily guarantee quality (or restorative) sleep. Restorative sleep is characterized by feeling restful and refreshed upon arising in the morning. Poor-quality sleep causes you to feel tired, achy, and irritable, even after an adequate number of hours spent sleeping.

Quality sleep can be precluded by such factors as changes in time zone and physical activity level, the use of prescription and illicit drugs, and nicotine intake. Anatomical structures such as large tonsils, a small throat, and excess fat around the neck can affect sleep quality by causing sleep apnea, a troubling medical condition characterized by extended periods of stoppage of breathing during sleep.

The best antidote for sleep disturbance is to maintain a regular sleep-wake schedule: that is, go to bed and wake up at the same time every day, even on weekends. Make sure you sleep on a quality mattress. Other strategies include eating a balanced diet and following a regular regimen of aerobic exercise. Also, you should allow at least four hours between your last meal of the day and bedtime.

If your headaches continue to flare despite a consistent sleep-wake schedule, talk to your health care practitioner about possibly undergoing a sleep study. Sleep apnea requires prompt professional medical evaluation as it can negatively affect your health in other ways, such as by raising your blood pressure to a dangerous level.

14. Get Rid of Social Habits That Can Trigger Migraines

Nicotine and the by-products of cigarette smoke can set off headaches in some predisposed migraineurs, as can alcohol. Some migraineurs can get away with drinking moderate amounts of alcohol; others have to abstain completely. Even if you don't have a problem with nicotine or alcohol, you should avoid using these substances as they can affect your overall health and can impair the efficacy of some medications.

Smoking and Secondhand Smoke Exposure

Nicotine in tobacco narrows blood vessels throughout the body, including those in the neck that go to the brain. This results in a reduction of vital oxygen, glucose, and other nutrients that nourish the brain. Smokers and bystanders chronically exposed to sidestream smoke can also develop chronic headache due to a buildup of carbon monoxide and carboxyhemoglobin in their blood.

Carbon monoxide, which makes up about 4 percent of the typical burning cigarette, aggressively dislodges oxygen from its receptors (attachments), leading to a higher level of blood carbon monoxide and reducing the amount of oxygen reaching the brain. Carbon monoxide also is a potent blood vessel dilator—another mechanism by which it causes migraines. Formaldehyde and the litany of other chemicals in tobacco may also play a role as migraine activators.

Kicking the smoking habit is very difficult for most people. Most long-term smokers are addicted to nicotine. The habit acquired from repetitive use and the purported psychological rewards further combine to keep the smoker hooked. Besides quitting "cold turkey," the best way to stop smoking is through a formalized tobacco cessation program that offers group support, and nicotine replacement and Zyban therapies. Most of these programs offer five to eight weeks of group support as well as instructions in behavior modification, stress management, and contingency planning.

The American Cancer Society and the American Lung Association recommend the following tips for breaking tobacco's grip:

- Set a quit date. Pick a date that's meaningful, such as your birthday or wedding anniversary.

- Tell friends and family members about your decision to quit. The aim is to get their support for your efforts and to help make you feel more obligated to succeed.

- Change your daily routine. Get rid of all smoking paraphernalia. Drive a different route to work. Refrain from sitting in your "smoking chair" while watching TV.

- Talk with your health care provider about getting his or her complete support for your efforts.

- Avoid tempting situations. Because smoking is not an isolated behavior (it is usually connected to drinking alcohol or partying), you may want to abstain from situations and events that may cause you to backslide.

- Learn a stress management technique, such as deep breathing or visualization, for dealing with the urges that are guaranteed to rear their ugly heads.

- Take it one day at a time. Remember: Learning how to smoke was a gradual, deliberate process; learning how to *not* smoke involves a proactive process that will take time.

Alcohol

Alcohol in all forms can trigger headache through multiple mechanisms, not the least of which are the migraine-provoking chemicals it contains.[31] Even nonalcoholic beer, which has no ethanol, contains these migraine triggers.

Alcohol widens blood vessels (which later narrow) throughout the body, reducing blood flow to vital organs such as the kidneys and brain. Some forms of alcohol contain sulfites, tyramine, and histamine that can set a migraine flare in motion by dilating blood vessels. Alcohol also containers *cogeners*, substances that give each liquor its color and flavor, which can trigger migraine headaches. The darkest alcohols, such as red wine, scotch, and brandy, contain more cogeners and are therefore most often implicated in migraine flare-ups.

Alcohol also causes hypoglycemia by triggering insulin production, leading to headache pain (see page 30). Bourbon, brandy, rye, gin, cognac, scotch, vodka, and whiskey are most likely to lower blood sugar levels. Alcohol is more likely to induce hypoglycemia if consumed on an empty stomach.

15. Use Medications with Care and Don't Use Recreational Drugs

Painkillers, diet pills, hormonal agents, and decongestants have been implicated as headache triggers in some persons with migraine headache. The drugs most commonly associated with headache are as follows:

- Indomethacin
- Nifedipine
- Cimetidine
- Atenolol
- Trimethoprim-sulfamethoxazole
- Zimeldine
- Glyceryl trinitrate
- Isosorbide dinitrite
- Zomepirac
- Ranitidine
- Isotretinoin
- Captopril
- Piroxicam
- Metoprolol
- Diclofenac
- Methyldopa
- Terfenadine
- Propranolol
- Benoxaprofen
- Metronidazole

Other categories of drugs associated with headache in nonsufferers include high blood pressure and anti-ulcer drugs, antibiotics, and antihistamines.

Painkillers

Some drugs can cause the very symptoms they are supposed to treat. For example, some painkillers effectively stop headache pain, but they can also *cause* headache pain, referred to as rebound headaches. A form of drug withdrawal, rebound headaches are a vicious cycle of chronic head pain/taking pain pills that goes something like this: the sufferer takes pain pills for a headache; as each painkiller wears off, the headache returns; this prompts the sufferer to take more pain pills; and the cycle continues. According to the American Association for the Study of Headaches, painkiller rebound represents the most common cause of chronic daily headache. These withdrawal headaches are similar to the caffeine withdrawal headaches discussed earlier.

Painkillers implicated in medication-induced headache include indomethacin, ibuprofen, naproxen, and other non-steroidal anti-inflammatory drugs.[32] Additionally, narcotic painkillers such as codeine, hydrocodone, oxycodone, and meperidine can induce rebound headaches. Rebound headache is best treated by withdrawing the offending pain medication and, if needed, using another type of analgesic — under physician supervision.

Diet Pills

The active ingredient in most appetite suppressants, both prescription and nonprescription, is either amphetamines or caffeine. Although the exact mechanism is unclear, many migraine sufferers report a correlation between taking diet pills and activation of their headaches. Caffeine-containing diet pills can set off chronic daily headache, forcing the individual to use more caffeine to counter caffeine withdrawal (see Caffeine on page 27).

Hormonal Changes

That 70 percent of migraine sufferers are women has to do with the hormonal changes that occur with menarche (a girl's first menstrual period), a woman's menstrual cycle, and the use of birth control pills. Indeed, the vast majority of female migraineurs first develop their headaches at menarche. The first menstrual period heralds dramatic physical and hormonal changes in a young girl's body. Menarche is a time of marked rise and fall in both progesterone and estrogen, the two major female hormones.

Oral contraceptive pills (also called birth control pills, or just "the pill") and other forms of hormonal drugs, and the hormonal changes during menstruation and pregnancy have been associated with migraine and other vascular headache. Many women develop their first migraine after starting birth control pills. The headaches promptly stop after stopping the pill. These headaches may be related to the fluctuations in hormonal levels that occur with taking the pill. I recommend that, unless the benefits outweigh the risks, you not take birth control pills if you have a history of migraine headaches or if you develop your first migraine after starting the pill. However, your physician is in the best position to help you make that decision.

After menopause, a woman's estrogen level decreases, placing her at increased risk for developing heart disease, hot flashes, and bone fractures due to osteoporosis. Similar risks exist after a woman's ovaries are removed—inducing premature menopause—due to pelvic diseases. The current recommendation for preventing these serious consequences is to replace estrogen and progesterone (referred to as hormone replacement therapy, or HRT) through daily intake of a pill or through a patch placed on the skin.

As with birth control pills, HRT causes migraines in some women. I recommend that you talk with your doctor if you develop HRT–associated migraine headache. Perhaps your clinician might recommend alternative strategies, such as consuming soybeans and soybean products, which contain phytoestrogens.

Decongestants

The phenylephrine and phenylpropanolamine contained in decongestants have been implicated as migraine triggers. These drugs work by stimulating the central nervous system and constricting blood vessels—two mechanisms that are likely to set off a migraine headache in susceptible individuals.[33] If you are a migraineur, you may want to avoid both prescribed and over-the-counter decongestants. Ask your physician if there are alternative agents that you may be able to take.

Cardiovascular Drugs

Cardiovascular drugs, used to treat high blood pressure and other heart and blood vessel conditions, have been blamed for migraine attacks.[34] As discussed earlier, nitroglycerin, an effective medication to treat angina, induces migrainelike headache in the majority of users, as do the blood pressure drugs hydralazine and reserpine.

Recreational Drugs

Similar in action to nicotine and caffeine, cocaine can significantly constrict blood vessels and trigger migraine headache.[35] In addition, studies have shown that marijuana can both treat and cause headache.

16. Learn About Common and Uncommon Types of Migraines

Prior to 1988, the various medical groups representing headache researchers and clinicians in North America, Europe, and elsewhere were unable to reach a consensus regarding migraine classification; that is, what names to assign the various forms of migraines. Regional terminologies such as "complicated migraine" and "migraine equivalent" had different meaning to different scientists, clinicians, and patients. In 1988, members of the International Headache Society agreed on a standardized glossary of headache terminology and diagnostic criteria.[36] The organization of headache experts identified nine different types of migraine headaches:

Common Types of Migraines

- Migraine with aura
- Migraine without aura

Uncommon Migraine Variants

- Hemiplegic migraine
- Ophthalmoplegic migraine
- Ophthalmic migraine

- Basilar artery migraine
- Abdominal migraine
- Status migrainous
- Migraine aura without headache

Let's look at some of the different types of migraine headaches and the events that characterize them.

Common Types of Migraines

Migraine with Aura

Previously called "classic migraine," this type of migraine is responsible for about 15 percent of all migraine headaches. The one out of six migraineurs who experience auras complain of a strange series of visual, motor, and speech disturbances prior to developing their head pain. Visual auras may produce flashes of light, or spots of different shapes and colors, or reveal only half of objects. Motor auras sometimes involve weakness or numbness on one side of the body. People with speech auras are observed to have slurred speech.

The aura phase of a migraine headache serves as a warning of the imminent onset of head pain. An aura typically lasts from ten to thirty minutes, after which the headache phase begins. An estimated 40 percent of individuals who have migraine with aura will sometimes have an aura *without* an accompanying headache, a condition sometimes referred to as "migraine equivalent."

Migraine Without Aura

Approximately 80 percent of migraine sufferers have migraine without aura, previously called "common migraine." This type of migraine usually lasts from four to seventy-two hours, is most often one-sided, and is commonly accompanied by nausea and vomiting. Sufferers report the pain as throbbing or pounding, and moderate to severe in intensity.

Uncommon Migraine Variants

Fortunately, less than 2 percent of migraineurs experience the uncommon forms of migraines, referred to as migraine variants. Most of these headaches are variants of migraine with aura.[37]

Hemiplegic Migraine

This uncommon migraine variant is more common in children than adults, and often there's a family history of similar attacks. During an attack, sufferers experience slurred speech and a temporary weakness or paralysis on one side of the body (hemiplegia) similar to a stroke. The hemiplegia may or may not occur on the same side as the headache.

Other symptoms of hemiplegic migraine include blurred vision and vertigo (sensation of one's surroundings spinning). These symptoms herald the onset, about ten to ninety minutes later, of a headache. As one can imagine, both migraineur and family members become very anxious during an attack. In very rare instances, the weakness or paralysis is permanent.

Ophthalmoplegic Migraine

This migraine variant is caused by dysfunction of the nerves that control vision. Like hemiplegic migraine, ophthalmoplegic migraine occurs most commonly in children. An attack is characterized by pain centered around the eye associated with a droopy eyelid due to weakness of the oculomotor nerve, enlarged pupils, and double vision, which can last a few days to a few weeks. Occasionally, the eyelid and pupil symptoms persist permanently.

Ophthalmic Migraine

This rare form of migraine, sometimes called retinal migraine, presents with visual disturbances that occur during the headache phase of a migraine attack. Sufferers report blind spots, total blindness, or vision in only part of the visual field. Ophthalmic migraine occurs primarily in young men.

Basilar Artery Migraine

Basilar artery migraine is induced by dilation of the basilar artery, the blood vessel that supplies blood to the brain stem (the base of the brain). Basilar artery migraine begins with loss of balance, difficulty speaking, double vision, transient blindness, poor muscle coordination, confusion, and, in rare cases, loss of consciousness. These symptoms usually last up to forty-five minutes and are followed by a severe headache at the base of the neck.

Basilar artery migraine occurs mainly among children, adolescents, and young adult women. Women sufferers typically experience this migraine variant during the week leading up to menstruation. Sufferers are at slight risk for migraine-related stroke. How and why this happens, and who is disposed to this migraine complication is unclear, although smoking and using birth control pills might be contributing factors.

Abdominal Migraine

This rare form of migraine also occurs mostly in children. Interestingly, during an attack, all the usual migraine symptoms occur except the head pain. Additionally, the sufferer experiences abdominal pain.

Status Migrainous

A rare complication of a typical migraine attack, status migrainous can last seventy-two hours or longer — sometimes weeks. Experts believe that prolonged inflammation of the dilated blood vessels is responsible for status migrainous. However, certain pain medications can trigger it. Sufferers are usually hospitalized to help combat the severe accompanying nausea and vomiting, and for rehydration (via intravenous fluids) and drug therapy to halt the attack.

17. Learn Whether Migraines Are Inherited or Acquired, or Both

Is migraine headache strictly a hereditary or an acquired syndrome, or a combination of both? Observational studies have revealed that between 70 and 80 percent of migraineurs have one or both parents with the condition.[38] But does this finding indicate a migraine-genetic link? Not necessarily; it can mean a common environmental influence or a combination of both factors.

Dr. Seymour Diamond, one of the world's foremost authorities on headaches, believes that the tendency for migraine headache to run in families probably is partly related to learned behavior, even though scientists have recently identified a gene that may code for migraine.[39] A child who observes the illness behavior of his or her parents might be attracted to the attention and special care that comes with a headache flare and thus emulate this behavior.

18. Understand How a Migraine Develops

Some migraine specialists refer to migraine as a *neurovascular headache* because one aspect of its development involves changes in the diameter and chemistry of the blood vessels (the tubelike plumbing) that supply blood to the brain and the nerves in the head and neck. Headache researchers believe that the pain of migraines occurs when blood vessels surrounding the brain become dilated (widen) and press on adjacent nerves.[40] Exactly how and why these blood vessels dilate is still a mystery, but it seems that some form of chemical signal activates the pain sensors in the trigeminal nerve that runs from a spot near the center of the skull up and over the eyes and toward the forehead. The stimulated nerve fibers release protein fragments called neuropeptides that cause the blood vessels to swell and become inflamed. The expanded blood vessels further irritate the trigeminal nerve—a sort of vicious circle—resulting in the head pain.

Another phenomenon in the chain of events during a migraine attack is activation of the pain center located in the brain stem (the base of the brain). Danish headache researchers have observed an increase in activity in the nerve cells across the top of the brain connecting to the brain stem of migraine patients. This spread of nervous activity appears to be one piece of the migraine headache pain puzzle.

Migraine headache also involves activation of certain chemicals. One chemical that has been commonly implicated in the migraine syndrome is serotonin (sometimes referred to by its chemical name, 5-HT), a potent neurotransmitter that helps transmit messages between nerve cells in the brain. Serotonin is normally present in the brain, blood vessels, and gastrointestinal system. More than forty years ago, scientists discovered increased levels of the chemical 5-hydroxyindole acetic acid — a by-product of 5-HT — in the urine of migraine patients at the onset of a migraine flare-up.[41] Current speculation is that changes in brain serotonin levels may also account for the nausea, vomiting, and mood changes that sufferers experience during a migraine attack.

A typical migraine attack has four distinct phases:

1. *Prodrome:* Fatigue, irritability, food cravings.

2. *Aura:* Vision disturbance (seeing flashing lights, blind spots); numbness or weakness on one side of the body; slurred speech; sensitivity to light and sound.

3. *Headache:* Lasts four to seventy-two hours. Throbbing headache (in 60 percent of cases, headache on one side of the head). Associated symptoms include nausea and vomiting, diarrhea, lightheadedness, dizziness, and ringing in the ears (tinnitus).

4. *Postdrome:* Fatigue, euphoria, surge in energy, increased appetite, confusion.[42]

Not all migraineurs experience all four phases. For example, people who suffer from migraine without aura skip the aura phase during an attack.

The Prodrome Phase

Some migraine sufferers report somewhat vague symptoms that signal the early onset of a migraine attack. This phase of a migraine flare is called the prodrome or preheadache phase. Some experts refer to the prodrome as the warning phase because it warns the migraineur of an impending attack.

Prodromal symptoms may precede the actual headache pain by hours or even days. Symptoms may include fatigue, mood swings, irritability, increased yawning, and food cravings.

The Aura Phase

Nearly 15 percent of migraineurs experience an aura prior to developing their head pain. What causes the aura and what actually happens? In most cases, the aura heralds an impending migraine attack, giving the sufferer time to begin taking a painkiller. Auras occur in the form of visual, sensory, cognitive, motor, or speech disturbances twenty minutes to an hour prior to the development of the head pain.

Typically, an aura involves visual disturbances, such as blind spots or flashing lights. Auras can also present with nonvisual symptoms such as weakness, tingling, or numbness in the face or on one side of the body. Additionally, slurred speech or the inability to put sentences together can occur.

Scientists now believe that the aura represents a brief constriction (narrowing) of the blood vessels that take blood to the brain before they dilate (widen). Migraineurs who experience auras show changes in noradrenaline activity that slows brain activity. The depressed brain activity results in reduced blood flow to some areas of the brain.

The Headache Phase

The headache phase of a migraine attack is the most terrifying to migraineurs. The head pain typically lasts approximately two to four hours, but it can last all day. It should be pointed out that migraines do not occur on a daily basis. However, a single attack may last for a couple of days in what is referred to as status migrainous.

The pain of migraine begins gradually and slowly builds in intensity. In about 60 percent of sufferers it is located on one side of the head. Sufferers describe the pain as sharp "like a knife" or a constant pressure that is located around the eye or in the temple area. Noise, light, and body movement typically worsen the pain, prompting the sufferer to seek a quiet, dark room in which to lie down.

Associated symptoms during an attack can include nausea and vomiting, dizziness, increased urination, and diarrhea. Some migraineurs experience pain in the hands and feet (likely due to changes in blood circulation), or tingling or numbness in the lips, tongue, or face, or in the fingers on the same side as the headache. Bystanders often report that migraine flares change the sufferer's personality.

The Postdrome Phase

After the pain and associated symptoms resolve, the migraineur may feel fatigued and listless and want to be left alone. (Unfortunately, this is the time when family and friends try to communicate with the sufferer in an attempt to comfort him or her.) In the postheadache phase, some migraineurs report a surge in energy, euphoria, and increased appetite up to twenty-four hours after the attack. Other postdrome symptoms include confusion, loss of memory, and clumsiness.

PART TWO

Migraines in Women and Children

19. Understand the Differences in Migraines Among Women, Men, Children, and Adolescents

When it comes to headache and headache triggers, are there hormonal differences between the two genders? How do these differences contribute to a migraine attack? Do the many hormonal changes that a woman experiences — menstruation, oral contraception, pregnancy, and hormone replacement therapy — explain everything? Do dietary patterns, physical activity, and emotional stress have major roles and, if so, where do they fit into the picture?

Overall, more women than men report tension-type headache (88 percent versus 69 percent), and approximately three times more women than men suffer migraine head pain. On the other hand, men suffer a sixfold greater incidence of cluster headache (a form of vascular headache) than women. Headache experts believe the marked gender differences in the prevalence of migraine and cluster headaches can be partly explained by male and female hormonal influences. Among women of childbearing potential (especially those in their thirties), the hormonal fluctuations during the course of each month provide the perfect backdrop for migraine tendencies.

During the prepubescent years, more boys than girls experience migraines; after puberty, the trend reverses — more girls than boys suffer from migraines. Authorities believe that the reversal in incidence is due to the difference in hormonal changes, especially estrogen fluctuations, that occur in girls compared to boys at the time of puberty. To be sure, medical scientists know very little about the biology of hormonal changes and precisely how these changes lead to migraines and other headaches.

20. Learn About the Menstrual Cycle and Migraines

Most female migraine sufferers, both adolescents and adults, trace the onset of their headaches to menarche. Dr. Christina Peterson, a neurologist and advisor to the National Headache Foundation, reports that the onset of menstruation is the single most significant trigger for female migraineurs.[1] Nearly 60 percent of female migraineurs who keep a headache diary are able to show a relationship between their menstrual cycle and their headache flares.[2] Menstrually connected headaches result from changes (either an increase or decrease) in the level of estrogen during the menstrual cycle. In a very complex relationship, estrogen levels directly affect the brain's endorphin and serotonin levels. As discussed earlier, serotonin, a major brain neurotransmitter, is responsible for the development of headache.

What's the difference between premenstrual migraine and menstrual migraine? By definition, *premenstrual migraine* starts from the seventh to the third day before a woman's period and improves or completely resolves with the onset of the menstrual flow.[3] Women who experience true *menstrual migraines* report recurrent head pain a week or so before the menstrual bleed, during the menstrual period itself, and up to three days after the menstrual bleed. Those who experience midcycle headaches are said to have menstrually related migraines. A small number of women suffer migraine attacks at ovulation, related to a midcycle surge in estrogen.

During the premenstrual phase of the menstrual cycle, water retention influenced by a rise in estrogen levels has an effect on the headache of premenstrual syndrome (PMS). Other symptoms of PMS include depression, fatigue, anxiety, food cravings, crying spells, cyclic weight gain, and breast swelling and tenderness. A number of theories have been advanced to explain the mechanisms involved in PMS–associated headache. The best explanation is that the widening of the blood vessels is triggered by hormonal fluctuations.[4]

Management of menstrual migraine is best started during the premenstrual phase of the menstrual cycle. The most effective treatment regimen for the headache is ergotamine (see page 116), avoidance of headache triggers, a healthy diet, regular aerobic exercise, and relaxation strategies such as biofeedback (see page 109). After menopause, when estrogen levels decline dramatically, menstrual migraines disappear or subside in most women. Sadly, a small percentage of women experience a worsening of migraines during their menopausal years, probably due to marked hormonal fluctuations during the "change of life."[5]

21. Learn About Pregnancy and Migraines

How does pregnancy affect tension-type, migraine, and other forms of recurrent headaches? Does pregnancy offer a reprieve from headache pain, or do headaches worsen during pregnancy? What are the mechanisms involved in headaches during pregnancy?

Pregnancy is a time of joyful anticipation for the expectant mother and her family and friends, but the majority of pregnant migraineurs report a worsening of their headaches during the first trimester, when estrogen levels rise dramatically.[6] What's more troubling is that the majority of migraine medications can't be safely taken during pregnancy. The good news is that 70 percent of headache sufferers experience a reduction or resolution of their headache symptoms during the second and third trimesters, when hormone levels don't fluctuate as much. Some women experience complete resolution of the headache pain for the entire nine months of their pregnancy, only to have a return of headache shortly after delivery.

There are many theories explaining the relationship between pregnancy and migraines. Why is it that some women experience improvement in their headache while others see a worsening of their head pain? To explain the reason for worsening migraines, one theory blames the escalating levels of estrogen during the early months of pregnancy, but offers no concrete explanation of how and why.[7] Other theories blame prostaglandins, hormonelike chemicals that increase the body's sensitivity to pain. To explain why headache improves in some pregnant women, some authorities theorize that endorphins, morphinelike painkillers produced by the body, may play a role.

After delivery, migraines are likely to return to prepregnancy levels, or sometimes worse. However, migraineurs who choose to breast-feed their newborns may continue to experience a reduction or temporary resolution of their attacks, probably because breast-feeding somewhat stabilizes estrogen levels. It should be emphasized that these headache patterns are not the same for all women. Even in the same woman headaches are unpredictable; indeed, a woman can have completely opposite experiences during two different pregnancies.

Because most drugs and herbal medicines are contraindicated during pregnancy, I recommend that if you are contemplating pregnancy in the future, you should learn to control your headaches through nondrug strategies such as biofeedback and relaxation therapy. Pregnant migraineurs should not use nicotine, alcohol, caffeine, and refined sugar—substances that may trigger migraines.

During pregnancy, your choices of safe painkilling and prophylactic drugs and herbal medicines greatly lessen. But if you absolutely need to take painkilling drugs, acetaminophen (Tylenol), acetaminophen with codeine, and meperidine (Demerol) are safe during pregnancy.[8] Women's health practitioners feel safe in prescribing the beta-blocker metoprolol (Lopressor) and the selective serotonin reuptake inhibitor fluoxetine (Prozac) to pregnant migraineurs who require headache prophylactic drugs.

22. Learn About Menopause and Migraines

For most women, menopause is a two- to three-year transition phase during which the biological ability to bear a child is lost. The biological events that characterize the "change of life" are marked by various degrees of hormonal and other changes referred to as the *perimenopausal* period. At the conclusion of the menopausal process, there is a drop and stabilization in the levels of estrogen in a woman's body. Similarly, premature menopause brought on by surgical removal of a woman's ovaries results in a drop in estrogen levels. Scientific studies during the past three decades have conclusively linked a drop in estrogen to troubling "hot flashes," emotional lability, and an increased risk for heart disease and osteoporosis (thinning of the bones).

As with pregnancy, different women react differently to the changes of menopause. For the majority of female migraineurs, increased headache flares mark the perimenopausal period.[9] Luckily for most women, menopause is a welcome relief because their migraine attacks invariably subside or disappear. For most women headache sufferers, fewer headache flares mark their postmenopausal years. Unfortunately, however, the drug treatment for postmenopausal "hot flashes" and other medical problems—referred to as hormone replacement therapy, or HRT—can mean a revisit of migraines.

Scientists are unsure why, like pregnancy, menopause affects migraines. The best guess is that the drop and fluctuation of estrogen levels during early menopause trigger migraines in similar fashion to the rise of estrogen levels early in pregnancy.[10] For some women, especially those without children or those who wish they had more children, the psychological state associated with the inability to bear a child may trigger headache pain.

Treatments of postmenopausal migraines include painkillers and prophylactic drugs, a balanced diet, avoidance of headache triggers, an aerobic exercise program, and relaxation measures, such as biofeedback or yoga.

23. Learn About Birth Control Pills and Migraines

Most birth control pills sold in the United States contain either a combination of synthetic forms of the hormones estrogen and progesterone or progesterone only. Also available are progesterone tablets and progesterone injections administered every three months, as well as progesterone implants that are placed under the skin every five years. Additionally, there is a morning-after pill that contains the estrogen-like hormone diethylstilbesterol (DES).

Birth control pills work by inhibiting ovulation. Ovulation signals the release of an egg from an ovary into the fallopian tube to be fertilized. Combination contraceptive pills suppress this process at the ovarian level. Progesterone-only pills and injections suppress ovulation by inhibiting the pituitary gland in the brain from releasing the hormones that influence the menstrual cycle.

The vast majority of women take birth control pills without any side effects. The most common side effect of the progesterone-only birth control method is irregular menstrual bleeding. However, for a few women, oral contraceptives can activate or exacerbate migraines.[11] These headaches may be related to the fluctuations in hormonal levels associated with the pill. DES can cause endometrial cancer in postmenopausal women exposed to the drug for more than one year. Female offspring of women who used DES during pregnancy are at increased risk for vaginal and cervical cancers later in life.

I recommend that, unless the benefits outweigh the risks, you not take oral contraceptives if you have preexisting migraine headaches or if you develop migraines after starting the pill. Migraineurs who smoke and take birth control pills are at increased risk of stroke. However, your physician is in the best position to help you decide which family planning strategy is best for you.

A large number of female migraineurs experience a reduction or cessation of their migraines after menopause, a change in life characterized by a drop in the hormone estrogen. However, the incidence of "hot flashes" and a rise in susceptibility to osteoporosis and heart disease that accompanies menopause cause doctors to recommend hormone replacement therapy (HRT) to their female patients. Like birth control pills, HRT involves using estrogen alone or estrogen in combination with progesterone to manipulate the hormonal levels in a woman's body for a specific purpose. The downside of HRT is exacerbation of migraine headaches. In addition, female migraineurs who smoke and take HRT are at some risk for stroke.

I recommend that all female migraineurs discuss the advisability of taking HRT with their clinicians. Ask your doctor if you might be able to control the effects of menopause via nonhormonal strategies such as proper nutrition (that includes soy products), regular aerobic exercise, and relaxation measures such as yoga and biofeedback.

24. Understand the Differences Between Migraines in Children and in Adults

A migraine is a migraine is a migraine, whether it occurs in a child or an adult, right? Well, not exactly. Although children suffer the same types of headaches as adults, childhood headaches are physiologically and psychologically different from those of adults. For example, children and adolescents with migraine headaches have auras that are slightly different from those that adults get.[12] In children, auras include confusion, hallucinations, dilated pupils, or difficulty speaking; auras in adults commonly are visual auras and involve flashing lights, zigzag lines, and bright spots of different shapes and colors. In contrast to the majority of their adult counterparts, most young migraineurs also experience headaches on both sides of the head. Children and adolescents also get more migraine attacks than adult migraineurs.

Migraine variants are more common among children and adolescents compared with adult migraineurs. For example, during the headache phase of a migraine attack, some children with migraine may experience severe abdominal pain (abdominal migraine or migraine equivalent) instead of the throbbing head pain experienced by adults.[13] The mechanism for this is unclear, but the outcome is that child migraineurs may be subjected to extensive and expensive testing to rule out abdominal disease while migraine syndrome goes unrecognized.

Diagnosing Childhood Migraines

The medical evaluation of children and adolescents suffering from headaches is similar to that of adults. There is no blood or urine test or x-ray study for diagnosing migraine headaches; they are diagnosed based on clinical features. Health care practitioners are trained to rule out secondary causes of headaches by taking a thorough history, performing a complete physical examination, and ordering appropriate blood tests and radiographic imaging. The signs and symptoms of migraine headaches in children and adolescents are:

Migraine Headache

- Nausea and vomiting
- Sensitivity to lights

Atypical Migraine Headache

- Slurred speech
- Temporary paralysis on one side of the body
- Vertigo
- Blurred vision
- Double vision
- Loss of balance
- Confusion
- Loss of consciousness
- Abdominal pain

Pediatricians, family practitioners, and other clinicians are trained to recognize the common clinical features of primary headache syndromes such as the aura, nausea, and vomiting that occur with migraines. They are also cognizant of signs and symptoms such as slurred speech, swelling in the nerves to the eyes, loss of consciousness, seizures, and fever that can signal brain infections and other forms of secondary headaches.

Doctors need all the help they can get when evaluating a child, especially a very young child, with headaches. An important role as a parent of a child or adolescent with headaches is to help describe your child's symptoms as completely as possible. In the case of a child with recurrent headache, you may want to help him or her keep a headache diary for a few weeks (see Appendix A.) In the diary describe what your child felt, where in his head he felt it, what time of day he felt it, how long it lasted, and what you or he did to treat the symptoms.

During the medical office visit, the doctor may ask about the family history on both sides of the family: whether or not parents, siblings, or grandparents get headaches and, if so, what type. The doctor may also ask about recent changes in relationships, school attendance, grades, or conflicts in school.

The diary will greatly help your child's doctor during the next stage of her evaluation. It will give her valuable clues during the physical examination, which involves looking into your child's eyes, ears, nose, and throat; listening to the heart and lungs; examining the abdomen; and evaluating the nerves that feed the child's eyes, head, and neck. The doctor uses the physical examination to look for clues, such as red eyes, that may offer valuable diagnostic information. During the neurological examination, the doctor may test your child's memory, evaluate his peripheral vision, check the sensory stimuli, and check muscle strength in various parts of his head, neck, and extremities. In addition, the doctor will check the child's reflexes and coordination, and his ability to sense vibration at the wrists and ankles.

After the physical examination, the doctor might order selected laboratory tests and x-ray studies, depending on what is gleaned from the physical examination. For example, if your child's doctor feels that a thyroid condition might be the cause of his recurrent headaches, thyroid function tests may be ordered to rule in or rule out this possibility. For acute headaches with features of a brain infection, a complete blood count and spinal tap may be done. If a brain tumor or blood vessel abnormality is suspected, a brain imaging study such as an MRI or CAT scan will be ordered.

Other laboratory and x-ray studies commonly ordered to evaluate children with headaches include chemistry panel tests, an electroencephalogram (EEG), and an electronystagmogram (ENG).

Treating and Preventing Childhood Migraines

As in adults, childhood migraines are managed with nondrug strategies and drug therapy. Physical activity can help relieve stress and contribute to overall well-being. Excellent examples of aerobic activities include biking, hiking, and swimming. Team sports are an excellent way for your child to stay active, as well as learn social and athletic skills and strengthen emotional and psychological health.

If your child is able to identify his or her triggers, such as foods, noise, or hormonal changes, help him or her remove or avoid the cause. For example, if nitrites are the offending agents, your child should avoid bacon, salami, bologna, and sausage.

If avoidance is not enough, medications should be considered. In the past ten years, there have been great improvements in the management and prevention of migraine headaches in children and adolescents. The discovery of some of the underlying mechanisms involved in the development of migraine head pain has led to the development of drugs that work to reverse the basic aberrations. Unfortunately, children and adolescents are not candidates for most of the newer antimigraine medicines. Pharmaceutical companies are currently studying the use of antimigraine drugs for children and adolescents. In the meantime, work with your child's doctor to select the most effective management regimen for your child.

25. Learn to Cope with School and Migraines

Children attend school to learn more than math, reading, and writing. School offers the child the opportunity to develop social and physical skills, build confidence and self-esteem, and learn to make the transition from one stage of life to another. Capitalizing on these opportunities is difficult even without distractions like a chronic health problem. Unfortunately, an estimated 10 to 15 percent of children with headaches miss school due to severe headache pain. In one study, children with migraines missed more than seven days of school a year compared with less than four days missed by their peers with other medical problems.

At the forty-second annual scientific meeting of the American Headache Society, headache scientists presented their findings of a study showing that up to 20 percent of adolescent headache sufferers (twelve to seventeen years old) experience migraine attacks on Mondays.[14] Conversely, only 9 percent of adolescents experience migraines on Saturdays. Lead researcher Dr. Paul Winner, codirector of the Palm Beach Headache Center in Palm Beach, Florida, felt that this headache pattern had to do with the anxiety of getting ready to go to school.

Indeed, children with recurrent headaches report a high degree of anxiety and depression related to school attendance. They are depressed that their peers consider them "weird," "different," "weak," and "undependable." Missing school, getting poor grades, and possibly flunking out add to the sufferer's misery. Anxiety stems from the uncertainty of anticipating a migraine attack with its associated disabilities, such as vision disturbance, difficulty speaking, and vomiting. Not surprisingly, many child headache sufferers miss a lot of school and usually lag behind their peers in schoolwork. What can parents, educators, peers, family, and friends of these migraineurs do to help prevent serious long-term repercussions?

A Solid Plan

Besides a thorough medical evaluation and treatment plan, young headache sufferers should aim to maintain the same social structure as their nonsuffering peers. Because there are widespread myths about migraines, educating peers, teachers, family, and friends should be a priority. Help them to understand the prevalence, effects, treatment, and prognosis of migraines.

It is crucial for the young migraineur to maintain maximum school attendance. Missing school due to prolonged illness, and not sharing in the activities of peers, can negatively impact a child's self-esteem.[15] Frequent absences can unintentionally reinforce "school phobia" and create a vicious cycle of headache-fear-headache. During an especially disabling bout of attacks, the child can still return to school for short periods of time. For example, he or she may return for two hours and gradually return to a full schedule over a ten-day period.

Another reassuring strategy is to develop a specific plan for dealing with a migraine attack. The plan should detail the following issues: who to tell; where the child should be taken during an attack; who will pick up the child and when; and what the family will do for the child on returning home.[16] After executing the plan, parent and child should jointly reevaluate its effectiveness and make any necessary changes.

PART THREE

Life-Threatening
Headaches

26. Learn to Recognize the Features of Brain Tumors

Many people with recurrent headaches worry that their headaches may stem from a brain tumor or some other life-threatening condition. Even migraineurs who've undergone complete medical evaluations for their headaches worry that a brain tumor is the source. Who should worry? What signs and symptoms are most often associated with a mass in the brain?

Although the incidence of brain tumors has increased in recent years, they are still a rare occurrence. The National Center for Health Statistics estimates that less than 0.5 percent of all headaches result from brain tumors. Interestingly, only 50 percent of brain tumor patients experience headaches, usually mild in severity, related to their tumors. Since the brain has no pain receptors, brain tumors rarely present with headache. In fact, less than 8 percent of patients with brain tumors report headache as their *only* symptom.

Tumors in the brain are most likely to cause seizures and disturbance in gait, vision, speech, coordination, and cognition. Headaches due to brain tumor worsen as the tumor grows, and are aggravated by coughing, sneezing, bending over, straining while using the toilet, or any other activity that increases pressure in the skull.[1] Brain tumor headaches are often worse in the early morning and can cause nausea and vomiting. Other reported symptoms include significant changes in personality, and numbness or weakness in the arms or legs.

I'd like to emphasize that only a physician or clinician working under physician supervision is qualified to make the definitive diagnosis of a brain tumor. If you're concerned about whether or not your headaches are caused by a tumor, check with your doctor or hospital emergency department at once. If your doctor suspects that you have a brain tumor, she or he will probably order a computed axial tomography (CAT) or magnetic resonance imaging (MRI) scan as part of the diagnostic workup (see pages 79–80). The treatment is surgical removal of the tumor followed by radiation or chemotherapy, depending on the type of tumor.

27. Learn About Meningitis and Encephalitis

Meningitis and encephalitis are potentially life-threatening infections requiring immediate physician attention. Meningitis is an infection or inflammation of the membranes covering the brain and spinal cord. Encephalitis is infection or inflammation of the brain itself.

Many pathogens, such as bacteria, viruses, and fungi, can cause meningitis and encephalitis. Viral meningitis is usually a self-limiting condition, rarely requiring hospitalization. Bacterial meningitis, however, can be a serious disease, requiring hospitalization and medication. Meningitis can also result from noninfectious causes, such as tumors and chemical irritation. Encephalitis, which can be caused by lead poisoning, is always a serious condition, with a potential for brain swelling, permanent disability, coma, or even death.

Besides a severe headache, signs and symptoms of meningitis and encephalitis include fever, nausea, vomiting, and pain and stiffness in the neck. Unrecognized and untreated, meningitis and encephalitis can quickly lead to seizures, coma, and death. Only a doctor or provider working under physician supervision is qualified to make the definitive diagnosis of meningitis or encephalitis. Most cases of suspected meningitis and encephalitis are worked up with a spinal tap (see page 82).

The treatment of meningitis and encephalitis varies, and depends on their cause. Bacterial meningitis, for example, is treated with antibiotics, while antifungals are used to manage fungal meningitis. Viral meningitis is managed via supportive care and observation. Encephalitis due to lead poisoning is treated with drugs that bind or *chelate* to the mineral, and steroids are used to decrease brain swelling.

28. Become Familiar with Ruptured Aneurysms

An aneurysm is a spot of weakness in a blood vessel due to thinning in the blood vessel's wall. This weakened area tends to bulge like an overblown balloon under the pressure of circulating blood. Over time, this aneurysm can burst, resulting in a sudden leakage of blood or hemorrhage into the brain and spinal fluid. If this happens in vital blood vessels, such as those that feed areas of the brain that control speech and coordination, sensitive regions of the brain are denied oxygen and other nutrients normally brought in by the blood. Eventually, this can result in a stroke or brain attack. In about 50 percent of cases, a warning headache occurs before the rupture.

Aneurysms rupture due to a variety of triggers, including severely high blood pressure, illicit drug use (e.g., cocaine), and strenuous physical activity. Symptoms of a ruptured aneurysm vary and can include a sudden, violent headache, often referred to as "thunderclap" head pain. Other common symptoms include slurred speech, confusion, weakness, poor coordination, stiff neck, and loss of consciousness. Obviously, a ruptured aneurysm is a medical emergency, requiring prompt physician assessment. Don't drive yourself to a hospital or have anyone drive you; dial 911 and ask for an ambulance to take you to the nearest emergency department.

29. Learn About Strokes

A stroke—a cerebrovascular accident (CVA) in medical terms—is a cutoff of oxygen and other nutrients to part of the brain resulting from interruption of blood flow. Medical authorities recognize two forms of strokes: one arising out of blockage of a blood vessel by a clot (embolic stroke); and one resulting from rupture of a blood vessel that causes a leakage of blood (hemorrhagic stroke).

Embolic stroke most often occurs when a blood clot breaks off from somewhere else in the body and travels to the tiny arteries that supply blood to the brain. If the blockage originates in the lining of the arteries in the neck and brain due to fatty deposits, it is called a *thrombotic stroke.*

Hemorrhagic stroke commonly occurs when the arteries are unable to tolerate the pressure exerted by the circulating blood. Two common types of pressure situations occur: an aneurysm unable to withstand normal blood pressure; and severely high blood pressure (hypertension) that, over time, causes the vessel walls to weaken and burst.

All strokes can cause headache, but the highest incidence of stroke-induced headache occurs among individuals suffering from hemorrhagic stroke. In addition to headache, stroke usually causes vomiting, and weakness and numbness in the arms and legs—symptoms similar to a migraine attack. As discussed previously, some migraineurs with aura are at a slightly higher risk for stroke, especially those who smoke and use birth control pills. If you are concerned about having a stroke, seek professional medical help immediately.

PART FOUR

Medical Evaluation of the Migraine Patient

30. Know the Details of the Headache Medical History

Your health care provider will likely ask the following questions about your headaches: How long have you been getting them? How often? What time of day do they typically start? Where in your head or neck are they located? What do your headaches feel like; to what can you compare the pain? How intense are they? How long do they last? What triggers them? What treatments have you received so far, and did these treatments help?[1]

Your practitioner may also inquire about associated symptoms such as nausea and vomiting, and whether or not your head pain was preceded by an aura (e.g., zigzag lines or loss of vision). If you have kept a headache symptom diary (see Appendix A), this is the time to review it with your clinician. The diary can be very helpful in identifying the type of headache syndrome you have and the headache triggers you're sensitive to, and even suggesting what treatment is best for you.

Because some types of headaches, such as migraines, tend to run in families, your practitioner will question you regarding your family history. Who in your family gets headaches and what type of headaches do they get? At what age did their headaches start? What treatments have proven effective?

Your provider will also likely be interested in the following: Are you married or divorced? Do you have children? Has there been a recent change in your financial status? Has there been a recent change in your relationships? How's your job, and how's your relationship with your coworkers and your supervisor?

Finally, your clinician will likely ask about your past medical problems to see if they may be contributing to your current problem. You should list any and all medical illnesses and surgical procedures you've undergone and the medications you are currently taking. Don't forget to mention any herbal supplements that you are taking, as some medicinal and performance-enhancing herbs negatively interact with some drugs.

31. Understand What Goes on During the Physical Examination

This is the hands-on portion of the evaluation where physical findings (e.g., a heart murmur) may offer clues as to what's causing your headache. The typical physical examination of the migraine patient may include the following:[2]

- *General observation.* This begins as you walk into the doctor's office. Your gait, demeanor, and overall health are carefully assessed.

- *Vital signs.* A nurse or other support person usually takes your temperature, pulse, respiratory rate, and blood pressure, and records them on your health record for the provider to evaluate.

- *Vision testing.* This test, also done by a support person, evaluates your uncorrected and, if applicable, your corrected vision. If you wear glasses or contact lenses, you will need them at this time.

- *Head.* The clinician examines the head to check for its general appearance, noting any unusual contours, tenderness, or rash.

- *Ears, nose, and throat.* The practitioner uses handheld instruments to look for signs of infection, sores, or anatomical defects such as a deviated nasal septum.

- *Neck.* The blood vessels, lymph nodes, and thyroid gland in the neck are evaluated via palpation and auscultation (listening with a stethoscope) for abnormal lumps and tenderness.

- *Neurological examination.* A complete neurological examination is vital to the evaluation of the headache patient. This involves a series of basic questions to check your brain function, and a number of physical maneuvers to check the integrity of your nervous system.

32. Be Aware of Common Laboratory and X-Ray Studies

Let me remind you that there are no laboratory or radiographic tests to diagnose migraine; any testing done is strictly to rule out medical conditions that can present with headache. If you've never undergone an evaluation for your migraines, your clinician may elect to order selected laboratory tests. These studies are usually obtained to rule out conditions, such as anemia, sinus infection, and thyroid disease, that can present with recurrent headaches. The typical laboratory evaluation of the migraine headache patient may involve a urine test, complete blood count, thyroid blood tests, and a general chemistry panel.

Radiographic studies are usually ordered to better evaluate unusual symptoms that can point to problems such as brain tumors or abnormal blood vessel pattern within or outside the brain. If the presenting signs and symptoms of your headache clearly show a pattern consistent with a primary headache syndrome, your provider may elect to forgo radiographic testing. For example, if you've had a migraine pattern headache for twenty years, dating back to your preteens, and your mother and grandmother also had headaches, chances are you have a migraine headache and a magnetic resonance imaging (MRI) scan isn't needed.

X-ray studies ordered for select migraine patients may include a computed axial tomography (CAT) scan and/or an MRI scan of the head and neck. Other testing done as part of a headache evaluation includes a positron-emission tomography (PET) scan, an electroencephalogram (EEG), an electronystagmogram (ENG), an angiogram or arteriogram, and a spinal tap.

Urinalysis

The urinalysis measures pH and the concentration of your urine output, and rules out kidney problems and other medical conditions that can cause headaches. Possible abnormalities found in the urinalysis include sugar (indicating diabetes), white blood cells (indicating a urinary tract infection), and protein or red blood cells (indicating kidney damage due to high blood pressure).

Complete Blood Count

The complete blood count measures the various components of the circulating blood, including white blood cells, red blood cells, and platelets. The blood count can detect conditions such as meningitis and encephalitis (indicated by a high white blood cell count), anemia (indicated by a low hematocrit), and thrombocytosis (indicated by a high platelet count).

Chemistry Panel Tests

This battery of tests evaluates the levels of a large number of chemicals in the body. The extent of this battery of tests varies, but generally the blood sugar, electrolytes (e.g., potassium and chloride), liver enzymes, and cholesterol are checked. The blood chemistry is ordered to rule out conditions such as low potassium (indicating tumor of the adrenal gland), high blood sugar (indicating diabetes), and high liver enzymes (indicating hepatitis) that can present with recurrent headaches.

Thyroid Function Tests

The thyroid gland, which sits at the base of the neck, helps regulate almost all bodily functions, such as the menstrual cycle, the rate of skin turnover, and the heart rate. Both hypothyroidism (underactive thyroid gland) and hyperthyroidism (overactive thyroid gland) can cause chronic headaches.

Computed Axial Tomography (CAT) Scan

A computed axial tomography (CAT) scan obtains three-dimensional x-ray images of the body by using a sophisticated computer-enhanced technology. Patients undergoing

CAT scanning are placed in a cylindrical tray over which the CAT machine traverses. In the headache workup, the CAT scan is used to detect brain injury that may indicate a tumor, infection, or stroke.

The procedure is painless and takes about thirty minutes. Some individuals experience claustrophobia while lying in the CAT scan's cylindrical tunnel. If you have a history of claustrophobia, ask your doctor to prescribe a mild sedative for you to take prior to undergoing the study.

Magnetic Resonance Imaging (MRI) Scan

A magnetic resonance imaging (MRI) scan obtains images of the body by scanning it in a magnetic field. Patients undergoing MRI scanning are placed in a cylindrical tunnel containing a strong magnetic field. The magnet interacts with hydrogen atoms in the body to create an image of various body structures. A computer converts the images into a picture of the tissue being studied. Sometimes a dye is injected into the vein to help "light up" the area being studied.

The procedure is painless and takes about thirty minutes. As with a CAT scan, some people may experience claustrophobia while going through the MRI scan's cylindrical tunnel. Again, if you tend to get claustrophobic, your clinician can prescribe a mild sedative to be taken ahead of time. You cannot undergo MRI if you have metal implanted in your body, such as orthopedic screws and metal plates, since these objects can damage the MRI equipment. Orthodontic braces can distort the images, but regular dental fillings pose no problem.

Positron-Emission Tomography (PET) Scan

A positron-emission tomography (PET) scan is used to image the brain's structure, activity, and blood vessel pattern. Individuals undergoing a PET scan are first injected with a compound containing relatively harmless radioactive isotopes that have an affinity for the various chemicals in the brain, such as glucose. The PET scanner measures particles called positrons emitted as radioisotope decays. A high positron emission from a part of the brain indicates increased activity. This study is used primarily to diagnose strokes and other brain dysfunctions.

Electroencephalogram (EEG)

The electroencephalogram (EEG) represents a recording of the brain's electrical impulses, akin to an electrocardiogram that records the electrical activity of the heart. The recording is obtained by attaching tiny electrodes to the patient's scalp. The entire procedure is painless.

Electronystagmogram (ENG)

An electronystagmogram (ENG) records the electrical impulses of the eye muscles. This rarely used study is ordered to rule out tumors on the cranial nerves located in the head and neck region.

Angiogram

An angiogram, also referred to an arteriogram, is done to evaluate the patency and layout of specific arteries, such as those of carotid arteries. This study is ordered to rule out blockage in the arteries. For an arteriogram, a catheter is placed in an artery in your groin and advanced to the carotid arteries in your neck. Contrast dye is then injected into the blood vessel to be studied and a series of pictures are taken to map out the architecture and determine the general health of the arteries.

Spinal Tap

A spinal tap, also called a lumbar puncture, involves placing a needle into the lower portion of the spinal canal to remove spinal fluid for analysis or to relieve pressure on the brain. This procedure is normally done to rule out a tumor or brain infection or if the spinal fluid is unusually high (as in a condition called pseudotumor cerebri).

Lumbar puncture incurs a slight risk of infection. After the procedure, be sure to lie flat on your back for about four hours to prevent leakage of spinal fluid. A small percentage of individuals experience benign headaches for days or weeks after undergoing a spinal tap.

33. Learn About Conventional Practitioners

Conventional practitioners are physicians who practice mainstream or technological medicine. In the United States, conventional medicine is practiced by two types of physicians: medical doctors (M.D.s), and osteopaths or osteopathic doctors (D.O.s). This differs slightly in other countries. In England, for example, osteopaths are not considered conventional medical practitioners and are regarded as complementary and alternative medicine providers.

Primary Care Physicians

Most patients seeking health care for chronic headaches consult primary care physicians. The majority of these patients have primary headache syndromes that can be competently diagnosed and managed by primary care doctors and nonphysician practitioners, such as physician assistants and nurse practitioners, working under a doctor's supervision.

Primary care doctors have a broad-based medical knowledge that also makes them good general medical diagnosticians and therapists. For example, their expertise allows them to recognize if a patient's headache stems from chronic sinusitis, allergies, or migraines, and to competently manage any of these conditions.

Family Physicians

In the United States and Canada, family physicians provide the bulk of primary care medicine. These versatile providers are well positioned to evaluate and manage migraines and other headache syndromes and to make referrals to specialists when indicated.

General Internists

Don't confuse the roles and qualifications of *internists* (doctors who specialize in internal medicine) and *interns* (recent medical graduates in the first year of post–medical school training). Internists or internal medicine doctors complete three years of post–medical school training in the management of a variety of illnesses, such as osteoporosis, heart disease, hypertension, and migraines. The training and experience of internists allow them to recognize medical conditions, such as thyroid disease and high blood pressure, which can present as migraines. Some general internists further subspecialize in specific internal medicine subspecialties such as cardiology, nephrology, neurology, and rheumatology.

Pediatricians

Pediatricians are trained in the primary medical care of newborns to children up to eighteen years old. Like family physicians, pediatricians provide a broad range of primary medical care to children. Their training and experience provide pediatricians with the expertise to evaluate and treat a wide variety of childhood diseases, including migraine.

Osteopaths

Osteopaths are physicians who are trained based on the medical model that the physical body, mind, and spirit are interdependent and inseparable.[3] Osteopathic physicians undergo the same medical school training as their allopathic (M.D.) colleagues, with additional training in manipulation of the musculoskeletal system. Today, most osteopathic doctors (D.O.s) practice in the same medical and surgical specialties and subspecialties as their M.D. colleagues. A few D.O.s exclusively practice osteopathic manipulation to improve range of motion, restore joint mobility and alignment, stimulate bodily functions, and increase circulation.

Specialty Physicians

Physician specialists practice in one or more narrow areas of medicine. With regard to migraine headache, both neurologists and headache specialists focus on this area of medicine.

Neurologists

Neurologists are general internists with additional training to treat diseases of the nerves and brain. Therefore, they are the most qualified headache doctors. Because neurologists have specialized knowledge of the brain and nerves, they can recognize uncommon conditions, such as migraine variants and brain aneurysms. Family physicians, pediatricians, and internists refer their difficult headache cases to neurologists.

Headache Specialists

Headache specialists are physicians whose practices are largely devoted to the management of headaches. Technically speaking, headache management is not a distinct medical specialty as is, say, neurology or endocrinology. Therefore, any physician can call herself a headache specialist. However, most headache specialists are neurologists, internists, and anesthesiologists. The obvious advantage of being cared for by these clinicians is their advanced level of headache expertise in evaluating and managing recalcitrant headaches.

Other Specialists

There are other specialists who care for patients with secondary headache. If your headache is caused by a problem with your vision, you may be referred to an optometrist or ophthalmologist. If you suffer from severe seasonal allergies, you'll likely be seen by an allergist. A general dentist or oral surgeon may be consulted if a jaw-joint problem is causing your head and face pain.

Otolaryngologists, commonly referred to as ENT surgeons, take care of ear, nose, and throat problems that can manifest as chronic headache. Finally, orthopedic surgeons and neurosurgeons evaluate and manage neck and spine problems, such as arthritis and ruptured disks in the neck, that can cause chronic headache.

34. Learn About Nonphysician Practitioners

Complementing the practice of conventional physicians are a large and diverse group of nonphysician clinicians such as physician assistants, nurse practitioners, physical and occupational therapists, and psychologists. These practitioners work with M.D.s and D.O.s to care for migraine and other headache patients. For example, family medicine physician assistants work with family medicine physicians to provide general primary medical care, including the evaluation and management of migraines.

Physician Assistants and Nurse Practitioners

Physician assistants (PAs) and nurse practitioners (NPs) typically practice under the supervision of a physician to evaluate and manage medical conditions traditionally within the domain of a physician. PAs and NPs are trained to take patients' histories; examine patients; order appropriate laboratory, radiographic, and other studies; and develop and implement treatment plans. These clinicians consult their physician preceptors for practice guidance.

Physical and Occupational Therapists

Many chronic pain sufferers report a reduction in physical strength, endurance, and confidence. These patients are often referred to physical and occupational therapists for adjunctive evaluation and care.

Physical therapists use heat, ice, special exercises, sound waves, and other means to treat disorders of the musculoskeletal system. For migraines, physical therapists use transcutaneous electrical nerve stimulation (TENS), a technique that uses alternating, low-voltage electrical current to stop pain by causing the production of endorphins. TENS has been shown to be an effective modality to stimulate inflamed nerve endings in people with recurrent headaches. Because TENS may interfere with pacemaker function, this treatment modality is contraindicated in people wearing these devices.

Occupational therapists focus on helping people develop proper physical dexterity and body posture to take on difficult day-to-day tasks at work and at home.

Psychologists

Psychologists are nonphysician mental health practitioners who are trained to evaluate and manage mental, emotional, and behavioral disorders without drugs. Psychologists employ individual and group psychotherapy to treat conditions such as anxiety, anger, and depression — conditions that can present with chronic headaches. These practitioners use screening testing to determine underlying conditions such as personality disorders. They also teach self-improvement skills and mind/body strategies such as stress management, biofeedback, and creative visualization.

35. Learn About Complementary and Alternative Medicine Practitioners

The practice of alternative medicine, sometimes called complementary and alternative medicine (CAM), is the fastest-growing segment of health care delivery in North America. In fact, 50 percent of Americans who consult conventional medical providers admit to seeking care from CAM practitioners. CAM refers to a broad range of healing philosophies, approaches, and therapies that conventional medicine practitioners don't use. CAM practices include the use of medicinal herbs, therapeutic massage, and homeopathy.

CAM practitioners who treat headache patients include chiropractors, acupuncturists, homeopaths, naturopaths, and massage therapists. Physicians and other conventional practitioners in the United States and Canada are gradually but steadily warming to chiropractic, acupuncture, homeopathy, naturopathy, and massage therapy as legitimate primary and adjunctive treatments for migraines and other ailments.

Patients who submit to CAM rave about its effectiveness, and more and more people are seeking the services of CAM practitioners. In 1997, Americans spent an estimated $27 billion on CAM therapies, more than the out-of-pocket expense for all U.S. hospitalizations.[4] For more information on CAM therapies contact the National Center for Complementary and Alternative Medicine of the National Institutes of Health (see Appendix B).

Chiropractors

Chiropractic medicine is now the most commonly used CAM therapy in the United States and Canada. Chiropractic was founded upon the belief that most types of pain are caused by dislocation of the vertebrae and joints. Accordingly, chiropractors employ spinal manipulation called *adjustments,* pressure, massage, and other maneuvers and use special devices to restore the spinal vertebrae to their normal alignment. They also prescribe nutrition and exercise regimens to help restore spinal health.

Chiropractors take medical histories, perform physical examinations, and order x-rays to diagnose medical problems. These practitioners evaluate and manage a large variety of musculoskeletal conditions, such as low-back pain, hip pain, and headaches related to malalignment of the spine.

Acupuncturists

Acupuncture has an ancient lineage, having originated in China over five thousand years ago. Ancient Asian medicine practitioners believed that a life-force energy, *chi* (in Chinese) or *ki* (in Japanese), controls the human body and protects it from disease. Opposing body forces, called *yin* and *yang,* must be in balance before *chi* can flow smoothly to ensure good physical, emotional, and spiritual health.

The premise of acupuncture is that life-force energy flows from head to toe via lines or meridians, with energy access points, called *tsubos,* to each meridian. The smooth bioenergy flow through the meridians can sometimes become blocked due to stress or muscle tension. Acupuncturists insert very thin needles in select access points for fifteen to forty minutes to remove blockage in the meridians and reestablish the free flow of *chi.*

After a century of waning popularity, acupuncture has begun to make a comeback in the West in recent years. Indeed, the American Medical Association, the National

Institutes of Health, and the World Health Organization have endorsed acupuncture as a legitimate form of treatment for a wide array of illnesses, including low-back pain, postoperative dental pain, osteoarthritis, and the pain of migraine headaches.

Acupuncturists, many of whom are licensed physicians, are certified to practice in all fifty states and the District of Columbia, and see over twelve million patients each year for a variety of ailments ranging from irritable bowels to migraine headaches. Acupuncture might be an effective adjunct or primary treatment for your migraines. Very rare cases of adverse effects from acupuncture do occur. Before seeking the care of an acupuncturist, check with your primary care provider to see if you are a candidate for this popular form of CAM therapy.

Acupressurists

Acupressure, also known as shiatsu, uses the same ancient Chinese premise as acupuncture. However, instead of needles, acupressurists use their fingertips, palms, elbows, knees, and feet to stimulate the acupuncture points to produce the same results as acupuncture.

This modality has been successfully used to treat various types of headaches, including migraines. Most individuals can easily learn to perform pressure point self-treatment with little instruction. To relieve headache pain, the following acupressure points are manipulated: the temples; the base of the skull, to the right and left of the spinal column; and the web space between the thumb and index finger. Additional acupressure points include the top of the foot between the big and middle toes; the area outside the shinbone, just below the knee; and the Achilles tendon.

There are many books on the subject, but it is best to first consult an acupressurist. Check with your doctor or other health care practitioner for a listing of acupressurists in your area.

Homeopaths

Introduced in the United States by charismatic German physician Dr. Samuel Hahnemann in the early 1800s, homeopathy became a popular form of therapy among American physicians. Indeed, at the turn of the twentieth century, more than one-quarter of all conventional physicians practiced homeopathy, and there were twenty-two homeopathic schools in large cities such as Philadelphia and Chicago.

Homeopathy gave way to technological medicine during the early twentieth century with the discovery and widespread use of antibiotics. By the mid-1940s, the practice of homeopathy was all but abandoned. In recent years, however, homeopathy has made a modest comeback in the United States, practiced mostly by medical doctors (M.D.s) and naturopathic doctors (N.D.s). Based on the "law of similars" where "like cures like," homeopaths believe that a substance that produces a certain set of symptoms in a healthy person has the power to cure a sick person manifesting similar symptoms.

Homeopathic practitioners use a variety of substances derived from flowers, roots, berries, snake venom, and other sources to relieve epilepsy, diabetes, headache pain, and other conditions. Homeopaths prescribe very diluted preparations that cause the same symptoms about which the patient complains. The active substance is diluted hundreds of times, with the quantity remaining in the solution being so small that it is actually submolecular. For example, belladonna, which normally causes a slight headache, is very effective in treating migraine headaches when diluted many hundred times.

That homeopathic treatments work defies all the conventional laws of medicine and physics. Yet numerous studies and anecdotal accounts indicate that homeopathy's effectiveness has to do with more than the placebo effect. Indeed, homeopathy has been shown to be superior to a number of conventional treatments. While medical scientists work to unravel the mystery of how homeopathy works and the extent of its application, migraineurs should check with their doctors to determine if they are candidates for this growing migraine treatment modality.

Naturopaths

Naturopathy is a system of natural healing employing spiritual, psychological, physiological, and mechanical methods, including water, fresh air, sunlight, heat, diet, and herbal therapy. Introduced in the United States by German-born, American-trained physician Benedict Lust in the late 1800s, naturopathy gave way to conventional medicine, chiropractic, and osteopathy during the mid–twentieth century. In recent years, however, naturopathy has been making a modest resurgence in the United States, practiced mostly by medical doctors (M.D.s), naturopathic doctors (N.D.s), and naturopathic medical doctors (N.M.D.s).

Naturopaths believe that the human body possesses enormous power to heal itself through homeostasis, restoring balance in the structure and function (mind, body, and spirit), and adapting to environmental changes. Naturopathy draws its philosophy from diverse traditional and modern sources. For example, acupuncture and herbal medicine are derived from ancient Chinese medicine, and massage therapy has a more modern lineage. Naturopathy is based on the concept that given the chance, the body will heal itself. Hence, naturopaths often prescribe diet therapy, regular exercise, massage, and psychological therapy for a patient so that her body can be stimulated to heal itself.

Naturopathic practitioners derive their remedies from plants, minerals, and animals, and from the patient's own immune system. For certain illnesses, naturopaths prescribe a twenty-four-hour fast with lots of rest and fresh water. Then fruits and fruit juices are added for a day or two before the slow reintroduction of regular foods. Herbs, vitamins, and minerals are also prescribed to help the body function optimally. In terms of safety, naturopathy has a good track record. The number of adverse effects due to medicinal herbs pales in comparison to the number of adverse events caused by pharmaceutical drugs.

Massage Therapists

Massage therapy, the manipulation of soft tissue, has been practiced for thousands of years throughout the world. Practiced by medical professionals, midwives, and shamans, therapeutic massage has been used to ease the pain of childbirth, sore muscles, and chronic headache. Massage fell out of favor in the West in the 1600s but reappeared in the 1800s.

Today, massage therapists are licensed in most jurisdictions to practice a wide variety of massage therapies, from the traditional Swedish system to sports massage and manual lymph drainage techniques. Massage therapists emphasize holistic health measures that include hydrotherapy, facial massages, skin exfoliation, reflexology, meditation, and aromatherapy. They use water, color, sound, light, aromas, and even herbs to appeal to the patrons' senses. A University of Maryland study showed that massage therapy was superior to some pain medications in relieving headache pain.[5]

36. Know the Facts About Chronic Pain and Headache Centers

When is it necessary to seek care at specialized chronic pain and headache centers? What makes these facilities better than general clinics? How do you get evaluated at these facilities?

The vast majority of migraineurs do perfectly well with care from their primary care physicians and CAM practitioners. However, a small percentage of migraine sufferers have headaches that defy the best efforts of primary care clinicians and neurologists. They fail multiple drug regimens, develop drug dependency, become depressed and anxious, develop musculoskeletal deconditioning, have failed relationships, and lose their jobs. These individuals are certainly candidates for specialized centers and clinics that provide a comprehensive approach to chronic pain management.

Chronic pain centers and headache pain centers approach recalcitrant chronic pain sufferers with the philosophy that multiple aspects of their existence have been profoundly disrupted—their jobs, personal relationships, self-esteem, and physical abilities, among others. Hence, the centers offer a multidisciplinary team of experts who range from physician headache specialists to physical and occupational therapists, registered nurses, and psychologists. Some offer acupuncture, massage therapy, biofeedback, and dietary counseling. Some programs are affiliated with medical schools and large medical centers with lots of diagnostic and therapeutic resources available.

Chronic headache centers do nothing but take care of chronic headache sufferers. This narrow focus brings to bear a high degree of headache expertise and also facilitates continuity of care. However, the biggest disadvantage of these specialized programs is that they are expensive, and care can run into the thousands of dollars. Some insurance carriers may not pick up the entire bill for such an in-depth evaluation and treatment of migraines. Because there are no national standards for staffing and equipping a specialized treatment facility, there is variation in effectiveness of these facilities.

Talk with your primary care doctor or neurologist to see if you are a candidate for a specialized chronic pain treatment facility. For more information, check with the American Council for Headache Education or the American Medical Association (see Appendix B).

37. Know What to Expect from Your Health Care Team

The clinician taking care of you should be your ally, advocating for you with all of his or her effort. You should expect the following attributes and services from your physician and other clinicians taking care of you:

- Complete honesty. Your provider should honestly tell you what he or she can and can't do for you. (And, of course, you should also be honest.)

- A complete appraisal of your health status. You should be afforded a full explanation of what your physical examination showed, all laboratory and radiographic studies, and any prescribed drugs.
- A reasonable amount of your health practitioner's time. As you may be aware, doctors and other health care workers are an overworked group of professionals. This fact notwithstanding, enough time should be allotted to allow you to ask your questions and get complete answers.

38. Get the Most Out of Each Health Care Visit

Because migraines can be a complicated condition, the evaluation process may take time to complete. Most migraine sufferers will end up making multiple visits to their doctors before a final diagnosis and treatment plan are achieved. There are no blood tests or x-rays to establish the diagnosis, so the evaluation focuses on ruling out other conditions that can mimic migraines and a trial of medications to determine the right ones. The following tips can help you get the most out of your health care visit:

- Prepare for the office visit. Learn everything there is to know about your headache. Write down all your questions before your appointment.
- Visit your doctor specifically for your headache. Headache evaluation is complicated enough, and being seen for multiple problems during the same visit will likely result in substandard care for your headache.

- Be honest with your provider about your symptoms, other health issues, current medications, and your fears.
- Be proactive during the visit. Take notes. Remember: The wise medical consumer is an equal partner with her or his health practitioner.
- Focus on solutions.
- Ask for detailed instructions on medication and nonmedication treatments.
- Follow up at recommended intervals.

39. Keep a Headache Diary

An invaluable resource in the success of the medical encounter is the accuracy of the information the patient provides the clinician. A doctor's evaluation and treatment plan are only as effective as the history provided by the patient. The medical history should include what, where, when, and how severe, and previous self-management measures and how they worked. The evaluation and management of migraine headache is no different. Most headache sufferers find it difficult to keep track of all the details of their disease. A missed headache detail can mean the difference between good treatment and subpar health care.

Most clinicians caring for headache patients would agree that the most important tool in migraine headache evaluation, treatment, and prevention is the headache diary (see Appendix A). Keeping a migraine diary will uncover a headache pattern and help your doctor diagnose the type of headache that affects you. The headache diary records the time of day the headache began; the weather conditions;

where you were when the pain kicked in; for women, the relationship of the headache to your menstrual period; and so on.

Remember, the best way to identify your migraine triggers is to keep a diary of your symptoms. Some migraine sufferers are able to conquer their migraines solely by avoiding their headache triggers. Unfortunately, others are clueless about their triggers and, instead, take expensive and unnecessary drugs to quell their head pain.

40. Form a Solid Provider-Patient Partnership

According to a study done by the National Headache Foundation, the biggest obstacle to effective treatment of migraines and other headaches is poor communication between health care practitioners and headache patients.[6] In the study, many physicians felt strongly that patients should educate themselves before coming in for each health visit to improve the doctor-patient interaction. Many prominent patient advocates as well as experts in health care delivery echo this opinion.

In our diverse and complex health care system, largely dominated by managed care, the success of the health encounter depends on the shared responsibility of the patient and provider. Partnering with your health care team is the key to successfully managing your recurrent headaches. Accordingly, managing your chronic headache is a collaborative effort among you, your doctor, and other health professionals working under your doctor's purview.

PART FIVE

Managing Your Migraines

41. Engage in Regular Physical Exercise
Regular Aerobic Physical Activity

As recently as twenty years ago, people with chronic pain were told to avoid physical exertion for fear it would exacerbate their condition. Impressive research in the past two decades has clearly uncovered the benefits of regular exercise for people with chronic medical problems, including migraine headaches. Inactivity leads to the following:

- Increased body fat percentage
- Poor muscle tone
- Poor digestion
- Poor sleep
- Low energy and chronic fatigue
- Low self-confidence
- A general feeling of "unwellness"
- Reduced bone mass
- Increased risk for injury
- Mental and emotional lability, including depression and anxiety

If you don't regularly exercise, you should set a date and start an aerobic exercise program after discussing your plans with your doctor. You should engage in moderate physical activity for at least thirty minutes three or four times a week. Regular aerobic exercise, such as walking, biking, jogging, dancing, and hiking, increases blood levels of endorphins, the body's natural morphinelike chemicals. Other aerobic activities include:

- Swimming
- Water aerobics
- Aerobic dance
- Basketball
- Tennis
- Racquetball
- Skiing
- Volleyball

If you suffer from stress, diabetes, high blood pressure, or elevated cholesterol, you'll benefit even more from regular physical activity. Other benefits of regular exercise include:

- Increased lean body mass
- Better muscle tone
- Improved digestion
- Improved sleep
- Increased energy
- Enhanced self-confidence
- Opportunity for socializing
- A feeling of overall well-being
- Increased bone mass
- Reduced risk for injury

Before you start, you should set a realistic goal. If you have been sedentary for a while, you should start slowly and work your way up to your desired fitness level.[1] Doing too much too soon can lead to fatigue, burnout, and injury. If you choose to walk, start with a moderately paced program for a few weeks before increasing your speed and distance, as tolerated. Progress takes time; be patient.

You should aim for an exercise intensity level of between 60 and 80 percent of your target heart rate. You can calculate your target heart rate using the following formula: 220 minus your age in years times 60 to 80 percent. Thus, if you are forty years old, you would calculate your target heart rate as follows:

220 minus 40 = 180, multiplied by 0.6 = 108
(if you use the 60 percent rate)

or

220 minus 40 = 180, multiplied by 0.8 = 144
(if you use the 80 percent rate)

Thus, if you are forty years old, your heart rate during exertion should be maintained between 108 and 144 beats per minute.

Anaerobic Exercise Program

How about doing isometric exercises? Weight lifting is an important part of any exercise program, but you have to follow the proper technique. Consider seeking the help of a personal trainer. If you have high blood pressure—especially if you are over forty years old—you should first check with your health care provider before engaging in isometric exercises.

Flexibility Program

In recent years, fitness experts have been mounting a campaign to get people who exercise to stretch and become limber before and after aerobic and anaerobic activities.

Flexibility exercises are just as important to health and well-being as running or lifting weights. These exercises increase blood flow to muscles and connective tissues prior to engaging in physically demanding exercises.

Flexibility exercises ease the strain on your joints, ligaments, and tendons by increasing the temperature in these structures. Flexibility reduces the possibility of injury by preventing your muscles from shortening and tightening during exertion. A good flexibility program includes range-of-motion exercises of joints such as the neck, shoulders, elbows, knees, and ankles. Additionally, flexibility involves stretching the back, arms, legs, and feet.

Watch Out for Excuses

There are very few barriers to exercising, but many excuses. It's easy to convince yourself at 5 A.M. that an extra hour of sleep is more important than thirty minutes of strenuous exertion. However, the benefits of working out far exceed the value of that extra hour in bed. This fact must be kept in mind when the litany of excuses for not working out comes up. Common excuses for not exercising include:

- "I'm too busy."
- "It's wintertime and dark during the time when I can exercise."
- "It's raining."
- "I have a physical impairment."
- "I'm too old for that."
- "I can't afford to buy expensive exercise gear."

As little as 90 to 120 minutes of exercise each week is all that's needed. Whether it means less time watching television or talking on the telephone, everyone can find time to exercise. Walking at lunchtime is one way to get around the excuse of "not enough daylight time." You should have an indoor exercise program, such as a stationary bike, for days when poor weather prevents outside activity.

Age and most physical impairments are not barriers to exercising. New research indicates that healthy people in their seventies and eighties can safely undertake physically appropriate exercise on a regular basis.[2] Even nursing home residents can benefit from modest forms of exercise. An effective exercise program need not be elaborate or expensive. For example, walking requires only a modest investment in appropriate shoes and comfortable clothing.

Exercise Under Advisement

Aerobic and anaerobic exercises can be downright dangerous for certain people. It is always a good idea to discuss your exercise plans with your doctor. This is especially important if the following criteria apply to you:

- You are a man aged forty or older or a woman aged fifty or over.

- You have a personal history of heart, kidney, or lung disease, stroke, or diabetes.

- You have previously experienced chest discomfort, dizziness, or shortness of breath during exercise or strenuous exertion.

- You have a family history of heart disease before age fifty-five.

- Your blood pressure is 140/90 or higher.

- You are unsure of your health status.

If you have never exercised or haven't done so in a while, you should consult a personal trainer. These exercise professionals can develop and help you implement a customized exercise program. They can help you select the right type of exercise and to pursue your exercise regimen without falling prey to injuries.

42. Consider Physiological Therapies

Many migraine sufferers have benefited immensely from physical therapy, massage therapy, and other physiological therapies. (See pages 108–112 for a discussion of alternative medicine practices.)

Physical Therapy

Physical therapy traces its origins to massage therapy used for the rehabilitation of injured soldiers during World War I.

Today, licensed physical therapists use both hands-on and mechanical means to treat a variety of musculoskeletal conditions. Physical therapy aims to strengthen weak muscles, improve the range of motion of joints, increase body awareness, and, ultimately, treat and prevent acute and chronic pain.[3] For migraines, physical therapists use transcutaneous electrical nerve stimulation (TENS), a technique that uses alternating, low-voltage electrical current to stop pain by causing the production of endorphins.

For home-care strategies and body awareness, the physical therapist may instruct you to consciously improve your posture and do neck and shoulder exercises. Shoulder rolls take only a moment and can be done a few times throughout the day, even at work. Stand with your arms hanging relaxed at your sides. Lift your shoulders up toward your ears, then push your shoulders forward, down, back, and up again in big circles for five to ten repetitions. Repeat this motion in the opposite direction.

Massage Therapy

Massage therapy, which has been around for thousands of years, is a popular form of alternative therapy in the United States. Massage therapy encompasses a number of massage disciplines including Swedish massage and reflexology, among others.

Developed by Peter Ling of Sweden in the late 1840s, Swedish massage uses stroking, kneading, tapping, and rubbing to release muscle tension and pain, including headache pain. The masseuse or masseur uses oils to increase circulation, improve muscle tone, and bring about total body relaxation.

Reflexology aims to promote relaxation and energy balance through stimulation of pressure points on the soles of the feet, and on the palms and ears. Originating in China about five thousand years ago, this therapy was introduced to the West in the early 1900s by Dr. William Fitzgerald, an ear, nose, and throat surgeon, who applied these techniques to relax his patients during surgery.

Exactly how reflexology works is still a matter of speculation, but proponents believe that pressure exerted at strategic points reduces the buildup of lactic acid (a byproduct of muscle contractions that can cause discomfort in muscle tissue). Others believe that stimulation of specific points enhances the movement of energy to corresponding body organs to clear out congestion and restore normal function. For example, the heel of the foot corresponds to the sciatic nerve, and the kidneys are stimulated by a point in the center of the foot.

Reflexologists claim to be able to help a number of chronic conditions such as chronic constipation, asthma, and headaches. Your may want to avoid reflexology if you have a foot or hand injury or if you have a history of blood clots in your legs. You may also want to avoid reflexology if you are pregnant.

43. Try Mind/Body Therapies

Few would argue that the mind influences how the body functions. Unfortunately, the research in this area is sparse, and the little that we "know" is conjecture based on positive results. The mind/body therapies that are most successfully used to treat migraines include stress management, biofeedback, transcendental meditation, yoga, and creative visualization.

Stress Management

Behavioral specialists define emotional stress as our bodily responses to everyday events. These specialists will tell you that these events, called stressors, are not in and of themselves stressful. What makes these events stressful is *how* we react to them. For example, a series of traffic lights turning red when we are late for an important event is not necessarily stressful. The lights turning red become stressful if we sit there and fume and complain about how "these traffic lights are an impingement on my freedom." Therefore, stress has to do with our perceptions and reactions to life events.

Common, everyday stressors include poor management of one's time, deadlines, unrealistic expectations, and disappointments. These factors or events can conjure up negative perceptions that lead to negative emotions that lead to numerous changes in the body, including migraines. Headache is one of many symptoms that life's stressors have outstripped a person's coping resources.

Stress management techniques have been shown to be very effective in relieving and preventing recurrent headaches.[4] The following strategies have been shown to reduce the effects of stress:

- Time management
- Delegation of tasks
- Realistic expectations
- Aerobic exercise
- Practicing mind/body therapies such as biofeedback, transcendental meditation, yoga, and creative visualization

Biofeedback

Biofeedback involves using audiovisual techniques (e.g., a beeper or flashing light) to help a person see or hear various bodily functions, such as heartbeat, respiration, skin temperature, or muscle tension, which are normally under involuntary control. The person can then learn to consciously moderate these physiological functions through operant conditioning.

Individuals undergoing biofeedback are taught to use deep relaxation, self-suggestions, and other strategies to alter the body function in question. When the feedback light flashes or the beeper beeps too often, the biofeedback trainee must use the learned techniques to alter the audio-visual signals and thus the body functions being monitored. The intent of learning the procedure is that the biofeedback participant will eventually learn to voluntarily control his or her biological processes without the help of the machine. Studies done with headache patients have shown remarkable results, with participants successfully reducing the severity, frequency, and duration of their headache pain.

Biofeedback practitioners include physical therapists, registered nurses, and psychologists. Like any new skill, biofeedback takes a while to master. Your clinician can help you decide whether or not you are a candidate for biofeedback and refer you to a reputable, certified biofeedback therapist.

Transcendental Meditation

Transcendental meditation (TM) grew out of yoga and Zen meditation. The physiological changes caused by TM include a decrease in metabolism and increased production of alpha brain waves—the kind that predominate when a person is relaxed. TM involves sitting in a comfortable position and repeating a sound or word for twenty minutes, usually twice a day. The goal is to eliminate all distracting thoughts and gain a deep sense of restful alertness to calm your mind and body.

TM techniques can be used to manage insomnia, high blood pressure, and migraines. Don't be disappointed if you fail to achieve dramatic results with TM, as it is not effective for everyone. If TM doesn't effectively manage your migraine but does help you feel more relaxed, it is still worth the effort.

Yoga

Yoga, which has its roots in Hinduism and dates back to 3000 B.C., teaches mind-over-body discipline. The various schools of yoga aim to achieve union and wholeness through harmony and control. Previously regarded as an Indian religion or a cult, yoga is now as normal a part of Western daily life as jogging. Practitioners occupy the full spectrum, from homemakers to Wall Street executives.

Indeed, the practice of yoga has exploded in the past decade in the United States and Canada as more people seek natural ways to improve their mental, physical, emotional, and spiritual well-being and to treat chronic conditions. Yoga has been shown, in anecdotal accounts, to control high blood pressure, arthritis, anger, and chronic headaches. Other reputed conditions for which yoga is beneficial include stress, immune system dysfunction, and painful menstruation.

Yoga instructors, called yogis, teach eighty-four different postures, called *asanas*. An important objective is to learn to assume a given position that will improve your circulation, restore normal body alignment, and aid other bodily functions. Once this position is mastered, the student practices proper breathing techniques that fill the lungs. Next comes meditation, made possible by proper posture and breathing, that helps remove you from your environment and brings peace, enlightenment, and tranquility.

Creative Visualization

Thinking makes it so.[5] The human mind has a unique capacity to create positive and negative feelings out of thin air. This power of the mind can be harnessed to relieve headache pain in two ways: by achieving a sense of calmness and by influencing your behavior. You can use your thoughts to foster positive imagery, bringing you a sense of calmness that relaxes your scalp muscles and improves blood flow to them. Creative visualization is a technique whereby the body's internal healing mechanisms are elicited by your conjuring up in your mind images of pleasant events and objects.

Creative visualization has been shown to produce a powerful effect on behavior. When you think of yourself as a person without chronic disease, you'll behave like a person free of illness. For example, if you have migraines and see yourself without headaches, you'll find yourself relaxing, even during stressful times. You can develop your own imagery. Visualize a pleasant scene in your mind or think back to a happy event from your past. For example, recapture the details of a momentous gathering of family or friends: Who was there? What happened? What did you talk about? Like other mind/body modalities, creative visualization takes time to master.

This technique is best taught by a trained and certified professional. Ask your doctor to refer you to a health care professional trained to conduct creative visualization sessions.

44. Know When You Should and Shouldn't Take Headache Drugs

Are you a candidate for headache drug therapy? Should you take over-the-counter or prescribed drugs? Again, the best person to answer these questions is your primary health care provider. She or he knows your health history, current health status, and when nondrug therapy is no longer the mainstay of your headache management. Moreover, your clinician knows which drug should be tried first, when multiple drug therapy is indicated, and how to monitor you for drug toxicity.

As discussed earlier, some drugs can potentially be double-edged swords—causing the very headaches they are supposed to treat. Painkillers, for example, can effectively stop headache pain but can also cause rebound headaches. The American Headache Association reports that rebound head pain linked to painkillers is the most common cause of chronic daily headache. Rebound headaches are a vicious cycle of chronic head pain and taking pills to relieve it, as follows: the sufferer takes pain pills to stave off a headache; as each dose of the painkiller wears off, the headache comes back, prompting the sufferer to take more pain pills; and the cycle continues. Rebound headaches are a form of drug withdrawal headaches similar to caffeine withdrawal headaches. If you experience the following symptoms, it's possible that you may have drug-induced headaches:[6]

- The need to take headache pills daily or almost daily

- Headaches that awaken you in the early hours of the morning (as the effects of the bedtime dose wear off)

- Nausea, abdominal pain, cramps, diarrhea, sleep disturbance, irritability, increase in intensity of headache—all symptoms of drug withdrawal—after suddenly discontinuing daily headache medication

Painkillers most commonly associated with drug-induced headache include ibuprofen, naproxen, indomethecin, and other nonsteroidal anti-inflammatory drugs. Additionally, narcotics such as codeine, hydrocodone, oxycodone, and meperidine can cause rebound headaches. If you think you might be affected by rebound headaches, see your doctor, as only she or he can treat you for this phenomenon.

45. Learn About Headache Abortive (Acute Treatment) Medications

There is a wide array of antimigraine drugs available to manage migraine headache. Abortive, or acute treatment, medicines are taken to stop the headache pain in its tracks. Pharmaceutical agents used to halt an acute migraine attack include the nonsteroidal anti-inflammatory drugs, ergotamines, triptans, sympathomimetics, barbiturate and analgesic combinations, narcotics, and corticosteroids. For the nausea and vomiting associated with migraines, anti-emetics (antinauseants) are sometimes used. Each category of drug is unique in its mode of action, rapidity of onset, and side effects profile.

Nonsteroidal Anti-Inflammatory Drugs

Nonsteroidal anti-inflammatory drugs (NSAIDs) were formulated in the 1960s to replace the steroids (or corticosteroids) that were found to produce a number of unacceptable side effects. The NSAIDs relieve pain by reducing inflammation, achieved by inhibiting pain-mediating substances called prostaglandins. There are more than one hundred different NSAIDs on the market today. Some agents are sold over the counter and others have to be prescribed by a health care practitioner.

Over-the-counter NSAIDs include:

- Aspirin (Bayer, Excedrin, Bufferin, Anacin)
- Ibuprofen (Advil, Nuprin, Motrin IB)
- Naproxen sodium (Aleve)

Prescription-only NSAIDs include:

- Naproxen sodium (Anaprox, Naprosyn, Naprelan)
- Piroxicam (Feldene)
- Diclofenac (Voltaren, Cataflam)
- Indomethacin (Indocin)
- Ketoprofen (Orudis, Actron, Oruvail)
- Nabumetone (Relafen)
- Sulindac (Clinoril)
- Etodolac (Lodine)
- Ketorolac (Toradol injection or Toradol tablet)
- Celecoxib (Celebrex)
- Rofecoxib (Vioxx)

NSAIDs are typically used to manage mild to moderate pain such as from arthritis, joint sprains, and gout. They are very effective analgesics without the addictive properties of narcotic painkillers. The most common side effect of these agents is gastrointestinal irritation, manifested as nausea, diarrhea, and pain in the abdomen. These symptoms can be reduced or eliminated by taking NSAIDs after meals or with milk, or by taking the prostaglandin analogu misoprostol.

Two potentially more serious side effects of NSAIDs a bleeding in the stomach and ulcers, but these genera occur with long-term use of high doses of these drugs. T

of the newer NSAIDs, celecoxib (Celebrex) and rofecoxib (Vioxx), were developed to reduce the likelihood of developing ulcers and stomach irritation. NSAIDs are contraindicated in people with a history of bleeding disorders, kidney or peptic ulcer disease, or any form of gastrointestinal bleeding. Pregnant women should not take any type of NSAID, including aspirin. Toradol should not be taken for more than five days total. As discussed earlier, NSAIDs can cause rebound headaches with chronic use. Children and adolescents should not be given aspirin, to avoid the potential for developing Reye's syndrome.

The Ergotamines

The ergotamines, or ergot derivatives, relieve migraine headaches by narrowing the blood vessels to the brain that have been widened during a migraine attack. The injectable form of the drug works the fastest, within fifteen to thirty minutes.

The ergotamines include:

- Ergotamine tartrate (Ergostat, Ergomar)
- Ergotamine tartrate and caffeine (Wigraine or Cafergot tablet; Cafergot rectal suppository)
- Dihydroergotamine (DHE-45 injection; Migranal nasal spray)

Used incorrectly, the ergotamines can become toxic to the body, manifested by a group of symptoms collectively referred to as *ergotism*. The most common side effects of the ergotamines are aching muscles, nausea, vomiting, and rapid heart rate. The nasal spray can cause burning in the nostrils and a transient sore throat.

People with high blood pressure, hardening of the arteries, angina, and disorders of the kidneys and liver should not take ergotamine derivatives. Pregnant women, breast-feeding mothers, and children also should not take these agents.

The Triptans

The triptans, or selective 5-HT receptor agonists, bind directly to receptors on the trigeminal nerve, shutting down the inflammation and the transmission of pain. These drugs are specifically antimigraine; they work at the root cause of migraine headache pain. Available as an injection, oral preparation, and nasal spray, the triptans are probably the most effective treatment for migraine headaches on the market today. Marketing surveys show that between 70 and 80 percent of patients treated with these drugs experience significant improvement in their symptoms.

The triptans include:

- Sumatriptan (Imitrex injection, Imitrex tablet, Imitrex nasal spray)
- Zolmitriptan (Zomig tablet)
- Naratriptan (Amerge tablet)
- Rizatriptan (Maxalt tablet)

These drugs act quickly, the fastest acting being the injectable preparation. Like the ergot preparations, the triptans narrow blood vessels in the head and neck. The most common side effects of the 5-HT receptor agonists are nausea, vomiting, dizziness, flushing, increased blood pressure, fatigue, tingling in the hands and feet, and muscle weakness. Individuals with heart disease and those predisposed to developing strokes shouldn't use the triptans. Pregnant women, breast-feeding mothers, and children also shouldn't take the triptans.

Sympathomimetic Agents

Isometheptene (Midrin) is a combination painkiller and sedative. Midrin works by narrowing the blood vessels in the head and neck. It is well tolerated by children and the elderly and presents no potential for addiction.

The most common side effects of Midrin are drowsiness and dizziness. Persons with glaucoma, uncontrolled high blood pressure, kidney or liver disease, or a history of heart disease, stroke, or other problems involving the blood vessels should not use Midrin. Concurrent use of Midrin and the monoamine oxidase inhibitors is contraindicated. Pregnant women and breast-feeding mothers should approach the use of this medication with extreme caution.

Barbiturate and Analgesic Combinations

Barbiturates are used to treat both tension-type and migraine headaches. These agents are effective in the majority of people who take them. Like most painkillers, these drugs can cause drug-rebound headaches.

Barbiturates and analgesic combinations include:

- Butalbital, acetaminophen, and caffeine tablet (Fioricet, Esgic-Plus)
- Butalbital, aspirin, and caffeine tablet and capsule (Fiorinal)
- Butalbital and acetaminophen tablet (Phrenilin)

Because Fiorinal contains aspirin, its use is precluded in people with a history of peptic ulcer disease and blood-clotting or bleeding disorders. The most common side effects of the barbiturate and analgesic combinations are drowsiness, dizziness, paradoxical excitement, and shortness of breath. Long-term use of these drugs can lead to dependence. Barbiturates can interact with antidepressants and should not be taken with alcohol.

Narcotic Analgesics

Some narcotic drugs are naturally derived from opium. Others are synthetic agents that provide the same level of pain relief as the natural compounds. Narcotic analgesics work by suppressing pain signals in the brain and spinal cord. Narcotic analgesics include:

- Acetaminophen, propoxyphene napsylate (Darvocet)
- Acetaminophen, codeine (Tylenol #3)
- Acetaminophen, hydrocodone (Vicodin)
- Oxycodone (Percocet, Tylox, Roxicet)
- Meperidine (Demerol)
- Pentazocine (Talwin)
- Morphine (Duramorph, Roxanol)

Narcotics are very effective at aborting migraine attacks, but long-term use of these drugs can lead to dependency, addiction, and rebound headaches. Common side effects of narcotic painkillers include sedation, dizziness, nausea, vomiting, urinary retention, and constipation. People with kidney, thyroid, or liver dysfunction should not take these drugs. These agents can impair judgment and coordination. Therefore, you should not take narcotics if you drive, operate dangerous machinery, or are required to remain alert.

Corticosteroids

Corticosteroids, or glucocorticoids, are used to treat acute migraine attacks that fail to respond to other classes of drugs. These drugs work by reducing inflammation.

The corticosteroids include:

- Prednisone (Deltasone, Orasone)
- Dexamethasone (Dexacen, Dexasone)
- Prednisolone (Pediapred)
- Decadron injection

The most common side effects of corticosteroids are nausea, indigestion, ulcers, elevation of blood pressure, and weight gain. Over time, these drugs can also cause acne, glaucoma, cataracts, ulcers, diabetes, and osteoporosis. Long-term use of steroids can suppress the immune system, making the user susceptible to infections. Corticosteroids should not be taken in conjunction with the NSAIDs.

Antiemetics (Antinauseants)

Antinauseant drugs are used to treat the nausea and vomiting associated with an acute migraine attack. These drugs suppress nausea and vomiting long enough to allow the migraineur to take an oral antimigraine medication or medicinal herb. Antiemetic agents work by suppressing the vomit center in the brain. Because oral medicines are difficult to take when you are vomiting, the antiemetics are usually prescribed as injections or rectal suppositories.

The antiemetics include:

- Prochlorperazine (Compazine)
- Promethazine (Phenergan)
- Chlorpromazine (Thorazine)

The most common adverse effects of the antiemetics are drowsiness, dizziness, and blurred vision. Alcohol can worsen the sedation of antiemetics.

46. Thoroughly Study Headache Prophylactic Medications

Some chronic headache sufferers fail acute head pain management and require an additional class of medications to help manage their headaches. For these patients, doctors prescribe a wide range of drugs, referred to as prophylactic or preventive medications, used to relieve or reduce the frequency, intensity, and duration of headache flares. Additionally, prophylactic medications help headache abortive drugs to work better.

Exactly what constitutes failure of acute headache medication? The following criteria is generally used to determine when migraine prophylactic drugs are indicated:

- Your headaches persist despite the use of multiple acute headache drugs.

- You experience migraine attacks more than two or three times a month.

- Your acute headaches last for prolonged periods.

- Your headaches are severely disabling.

- You take drugs or have a medical condition that precludes the acute headache drugs.

- Your acute headache drugs cause undesirable side effects.

Migraine prophylactic drugs include the beta-blockers, calcium channel blockers, antidepressants, anticonvulsants, serotonin receptor antagonists, and NSAIDs. You'll notice that the NSAIDs are used as both abortive and prophylactic antimigraine agents.

Beta-Blockers

Beta-blockers are the most popular migraine prevention drugs.[7] They work by maintaining blood vessels at a relatively dilated and stable size. One event in the migraine attack cascade is instability in the size or diameter of the blood vessels that go to the head and neck. By stabilizing the size of these blood vessels, beta-blockers treat an important aspect of the migraine process. Beta-blockers are also used to treat high blood pressure, angina, and certain other heart diseases.

Beta-blockers include:

- Propranolol (Inderal)
- Atenolol (Tenormin)
- Metoprolol (Lopressor)
- Nadolol (Corgard)

The most commonly reported side effects of beta-blockers include fatigue, reduced exercise tolerance, loss of memory, and impotence. Beta-blockers slow the metabolism of some users, reducing caloric burning and causing weight gain. Persons who suffer from asthma and depression may also want to avoid these drugs, as they can worsen both. Pregnant and breast-feeding women should not take beta-blockers. Type I (insulin-dependent) diabetics should also avoid taking these drugs.

Calcium Channel Blockers

Calcium channel blockers (CCBs), also called calcium blockers, relax the muscles in blood vessel walls by reducing calcium flow into muscle cells, resulting in dilation of lumen of blood vessels. Doctors also prescribe these drugs to lower blood pressure and to control the heartbeat in persons with an irregular heartbeat. Migraineurs with aura seem to do better with CCBs than migraineurs without aura. Calcium channel blockers include:

- Verapamil (Calan, Verelan, or Isoptan tablet)
- Nimodipine (Nimotop tablet)
- Diltiazem (Cardizem or Tiazac tablet)
- Nifedipine (Procardia or Adalat tablet)
- Nicardipine (Cardene tablet)

The most common side effects of CCBs are temporary headaches (which is what they are supposed to treat in the first place!), low blood pressure, retained fluid, constipation, drowsiness, and weight gain. In the majority of users, these side effects clear after a few weeks of taking the drug. Grapefruit or grapefruit juice should not be taken in conjunction with CCBs as it can impair the enzyme responsible for breaking down CCBs. CCBs can block the electrical activity in the heart when combined with beta-blockers in people with a condition called atrioventricular block. CCBs may also increase the blood levels of theophylline and quinidine when taken together.

Antidepressants

Many headache experts recommend antidepressants in the management of chronic headaches, especially for persons with chronic daily headaches and migraines. Currently, there are four main classes of antidepressants available in the United States: the tricyclic antidepressants (TCAs), the tetracyclic antidepressants, the selective serotonin reuptake inhibitors, and the monoamine oxidase inhibitors.

Tricyclic Antidepressants

Tricyclic antidepressants (TCAs) work by increasing the level of the neurotransmitter serotonin in the brain by preventing its reabsorption into the nerve terminals. These drugs are ideal for headache sufferers with coincidental depression and sleep disorder.

The tricyclic antidepressants include:

- Amitriptyline (Elavil, Endep)
- Nortriptyline (Pamelor, Aventyl)
- Desipramine (Norpramin)
- Doxepin (Sinequan, Adapin)
- Trazodone (Desyrel)
- Imipramine (Tofranil)
- Trimipramine (Surmontil)

The most common adverse effects of the TCAs are sedation, dry mouth, constipation, loss of libido, and weight gain. These drugs should not be taken if you have a disturbance with your heart rhythm, have had a recent heart attack, or have a history of epilepsy.

Tetracyclic Antidepressants

Although no scientific studies have shown their efficacy in treating migraines, the tetracyclic agents work in similar fashion to the TCAs. Drugs in this class of antidepressants include mirtazapine (Remeron) and maprotiline (Ludiomil). The most common side effects of the tetracyclic agents are drowsiness, increased appetite, weight gain, dry mouth, and constipation. As with the TCAs, you should not drive, operate heavy machinery, or take other sedative drugs while taking tetracyclic antidepressants. These drugs can take two to four weeks to achieve maximum therapeutic benefits.

Selective Serotonin Reuptake Inhibitors

The selective serotonin reuptake inhibitors (SSRIs) work at the 5-HT receptors to increase the concentration of brain serotonin levels. In addition to depression and chronic headache prevention, some SSRIs are used to treat obsessive-compulsive disorder and bulimia nervosa.

The selective serotonin reuptake inhibitors include:

- Fluoxetine (Prozac, Sarafem)

- Paroxetene (Paxil)

- Sertraline (Zoloft)

- Fluvoxamine (Luvox)

- Venlafaxine (Effexor)

- Citalopram (Celexa)

The most common side effects of the SSRIs are insomnia, weight loss, reduced libido, male sexual dysfunction, and increased depression. These drugs are contraindicated for concurrent use with the monoamine oxidase inhibitor class of antidepressants (discussed next). The SSRIs may increase or decrease the blood levels of other drugs such as lithium, digoxin, theophylline, and phenobarbital.

Monoamine Oxidase Inhibitors

The monoamine oxidase inhibitors (MAOIs) are the oldest class of antidepressant drugs. They have significant side effects and interact with many other drugs. For these reasons, MAOIs are rarely used today. MAOIs are effective in managing migraines that fail to respond to other prophylactic migraine drugs. However, the side effect profile of these drugs and their potential to interact with many foods and drugs limit their use.

Monoamine oxidase inhibitors include:

- Tranylcypromine (Parnate)
- Phenelzine (Nardil)
- Isocarboxazid (Marplan)

The most common side effects of MAOIs include low blood pressure, headache, impotence, and drowsiness. MAOI users should not consume tyramine-containing foods such as aged cheese or red wine. MAOIs should not be used with tricyclic antidepressants, or antidiabetic and anti-Parkinson's drugs. Don't start MAOIs within five weeks of taking an SSRI.

Anticonvulsants

Anticonvulsants or antiepileptic drugs work by quieting the electrically irritable migraine brain.[8] These drugs are convenient for migraineurs who also happen to have a seizure disorder.

Anticonvulsants used to prevent migraines include:

- Phenytoin (Dilantin)
- Carbamazepine (Tegretol)
- Divalproex sodium (Depakote)

The most frequent anticonvulsant-induced side effects include nausea, dizziness, drowsiness, insomnia, weight gain, and hair loss. Phenytoin can cause thickening of the gums, especially in individuals with poor dental hygiene. You shouldn't take these drugs if you have liver disease.

Anticonvulsants may reduce the effectiveness of birth control pills. Additionally, these drugs are contraindicated during pregnancy.

Serotonin Receptor Antagonists

Methysergide maleate (Sansert) has been used in the United States since the 1950s to prevent migraines. It is a synthetic agent that is chemically related to the naturally occurring ergotamine medications. However, because of its potentially adverse effects with long-term use (formation of fibrous tissue around the kidneys, in the lungs, or in the heart valves), this agent is reserved for use by individuals with severe migraines who fail other preventive drug treatments.

The most common side effects of methysergide are nausea, drowsiness, dizziness, insomnia, muscle cramps, and pain or swelling in the extremities. Patients placed on methysergide to prevent migraines should not be kept on it for more than four to six months consecutively, and should be taken off of it for four to six weeks. These patients should also be monitored periodically to ensure that they don't develop fibrous tissue. Methysergide is contraindicated in patients with a history of collagen disease (e.g., lupus), severe high blood pressure, coronary heart disease, and blood clots.

Other Migraine Prophylactic Agents

In addition to their use during acute flare-ups, methysergide and the NSAIDs are also prescribed as migraine prophylactic agents. Cyproheptadine (Periactin), an antihistamine (to treat hay fever and hives) with a chemical structure similar to that of the TCAs, is occasionally used to reduce the frequency, severity, and duration of migraines.

Periactin can cause sedation, increased appetite, weight gain, dizziness, and dry mouth. Interestingly, children seem to tolerate Periactin better than do adults.

Clonidine (Catapress), a centrally acting alpha-blocker normally used to treat high blood pressure and other cardiovascular conditions, is sometimes used to reduce the frequency, severity, and duration of migraines. This drug is as effective as the beta-blockers in migraine prophylaxis. The most common side effects of clonidine are dry mouth, constipation, dizziness, drowsiness, and depression.

47. Become Familiar with Migraine Medicinal Herbs

The use of medicinal herbs in the treatment of acute and chronic conditions is not such a revolutionary idea; it's been around for thousands of years in Asia and Europe. What we now call complementary and alternative medicine (CAM) in the West, which includes herbal therapy, used to be mainstream medicine but was pushed aside in the eighteenth century in favor of scientific, or contemporary, medicine. Unlike conventional drugs, some CAM treatments have not been subjected to the strictest of scientific scrutiny. But does this mean that CAM therapies are useless?

In the past ten years, the use of herbs has been making a steady comeback in the United States and Canada. In 2000, Americans spent an estimated $14 billion on medicinal herbs and other dietary supplements, up from $6.5 billion in 1996 and $3.3 billion in 1990.[9] Surveys have shown that more than 50 percent of all Americans take dietary supplements regularly.[10] People are drawn to the fact that these agents are marketed as natural products and referred to as dietary supplements. Many users of herbal products extol the virtues of these agents. New herbal distribution outlets are springing up everywhere, from Wall Street to Main Street.

Nevertheless, when it comes to the manufacture, sale, and consumption of supplement products, there is no shortage of critics and defenders. Critics of the dietary supplement industry charge that there is relatively poor federal regulatory oversight of herbal and other supplements despite the fact that they possess powerful druglike properties. On the other hand, proponents of dietary supplements point out that these products have been used in Europe and Asia for centuries, and that in some countries the use of medicinal herbs has eclipsed that of pharmaceutical drugs. In Germany, for instance, conventionally trained physicians are required to have training in herbal medicine. In terms of safety, the number of adverse effects caused by medicinal herbs pales in comparison to those caused by pharmaceutical drugs.

Herbal agents that have shown efficacy in treating migraine headache include feverfew, valerian root, ginger root, and Jamaican dogwood. Like pharmaceutical drugs, some medicinal herbs are best suited to halt acute attacks while others are prophylactic agents. However, the lines of demarcation of abortive versus prophylactic agents are not as clear with medicinal herbs as they are with regular drugs.

Some herbal agents are metabolized by the same body organs (e.g., the liver) as pharmaceutical drugs are. This can lead to a potentially dangerous herb-drug interaction. That these products are natural doesn't mean that you can take as many as you want; they have as many pharmacological restrictions (e.g., dosage and side effects) as regular drugs.

Additionally, the contraindications for some of these agents (e.g., don't take if you are pregnant) have not been clearly established. My recommendation is not to take any herbal products on a short-term or long-term basis before consulting your headache doctor or a qualified herbalist.

Feverfew (*Tanacetum parthenium*)

Feverfew has been used extensively in Europe for centuries and has been shown in several studies to reduce the severity and frequency of migraines.[11] Derived from a plant in the chrysanthemum family, this agent was used in medieval Europe to treat fever and headache.[12] It is also a relaxant, a blood vessel dilator (enlarging the diameter by relaxing the walls), and a uterine stimulant.

Feverfew is available in a capsule or as a tincture for the prevention of migraines. As a prophylactic migraine agent, it isn't effective in treating or aborting acute headache pain. Maximum efficacy may take several weeks. The most common side effects of this herb are nausea, mouth ulcers, lip swelling, loss of taste, and rash. Pregnant women should not take feverfew because it is a uterine stimulant. Breast-feeding women should refrain from taking this herb as its safety for children under two years of age has not been established. Take this agent only under the supervision of your doctor or herbalist.

Valerian (*Valeriana officinalis*)

Valerian dates back to medieval times when the Greeks used it to treat digestive problems such as nausea and gas. Over the centuries, its use has varied from treating menstrual cramps to panic disorder.

More recently, valerian has been shown to be effective in relieving mild insomnia, bronchial spasm, and migraine headaches. It can be taken as a tea or tincture, and can be mixed with other herbs to treat coincidental conditions. This herb may be toxic in high doses and may cause headaches, insomnia, and agitation with prolonged use. Pregnant women should not take valerian. Check with your doctor or herbalist before taking this herb.

White Willow Bark (*Salix alba*)

White willow bark contains natural salicylates with a chemical structure similar to that of aspirin. Like aspirin, white willow bark is an anti-inflammatory, analgesic, and fever reducer. Unlike aspirin, however, white willow bark is less likely to induce stomach upset and gastrointestinal bleeding. For centuries, willow bark tea was—and still is—a folk remedy for fever and pain among American Indians and Europeans.

White willow bark very effectively relieves the pain of migraine headache. Unlike narcotic painkillers, it is not habit-forming and doesn't cause sedation. White willow bark can be taken with other herbal pain relievers. It comes as a capsule, tincture, and tea. This agent should be taken under the supervision of your doctor or herbalist.

Skullcap (*Scutellaria lateriflora*)

A member of the mint family, skullcap has been used in combination with valerian as a mild sedative. Researchers have uncovered scant evidence that skullcap lowers blood pressure, reduces irritability and restlessness, and relieves flu symptoms. Skullcap can be purchased as a tea, tincture, or capsule. It is very safe, but cases of damage to the liver have been reported. This herb should only be taken under the supervision of a competent health care professional.

Ginger (*Zingiber officinale*)

Regular household ginger has many uses, such as lowering cholesterol, preventing seasickness, and helping digestion. Its anti–nausea/vomiting properties and its ability to inhibit platelet clumping make it effective for the treatment of migraine headaches. Ginger root tea can be steeped or boiled. Ginger is also available as a tincture, a powder, and in tablet form. No toxicity has been reported with ginger, but pregnant women should avoid this herb.[13] Migraineurs should check with their doctors or herbalists before using ginger to manage migraine headaches.

Jamaican Dogwood (*Piscidia erythrina*)

Jamaican dogwood can be used in managing insomnia and neuralgia. It can also be used to treat acute migraine flare-ups, as well as to prevent migraine attacks.[14] Jamaican dogwood can be used to make a tea or can be purchased as a tablet. Although there are very few cases of toxicity, it should be remembered that this is a potent herb and exceeding the recommended dosage can cause nausea, vomiting, convulsions, and a drop in blood pressure. Take Jamaican dogwood only with the approval of your doctor or a qualified herbalist.

St. John's Wort (*Hypericum perforatum*)

One of the most popular herbs sold in the United States and Canada, St. John's wort has been touted as being very effective in relieving mild depression. In Germany, it is prescribed more often than Prozac for mild depression. This herb has been around a long time, dating back before the

Middle Ages. The Greeks and Romans carried it around to ward off evil spirits. Studies have shown that St. John's wort is also effective for treating migraines.

The herb can be used to make a tea or can be purchased as a tablet. Although there are very few cases of toxicity, St. John's wort can cause sunburn in some people. Potential side effects include urinary retention, indigestion, and fatigue. There are a number of known drug-herb interactions between St. John's wort and Prozac, other antidepressants, digoxin, Buspar, Cardizem, and Viagra, to name a few. Take St. John's wort only under your doctor's or herbalist's supervision.

48. Calculate the Financial Impact of Your Headache

The cost of preventing and treating chronic headaches can quickly add up. Migraine headaches cost employers and patients a whopping $11 billion annually. Some employers pay out well over $5,000 a year in health premiums for each employee who suffers from chronic headaches. Individual consumers spend an additional $4 billion on over-the-counter painkillers. And let's not forget to mention the multiple billions wasted on products hawked by charlatans.

In today's complex health care market, consumers are faced with many daunting issues, such as dealing with insurance companies and managed-care organizations, and paying for the high cost of prescription and nonprescription drugs. Those who do their homework and learn about the intricacies of the marketplace come out ahead. As a consumer of health care services and products, you owe it to yourself to get the best deal for your hard-earned money.

Appendix B lists the addresses of many agencies and organizations that serve as information clearinghouses for all types of consumer goods and services.

49. Be Sure You Have Health Insurance Coverage

Migraine sufferers are at a tremendous disadvantage when it comes to getting health insurance coverage.[15] Not only is their condition expensive to evaluate and treat, but insurance companies also make it difficult to collect on claims. Since there are no blood tests or x-rays to specifically diagnose migraines and testing is usually done to rule out other conditions that can mimic migraines, health insurers invariably question physicians' medical evaluations of headache patients. So how can you get the care you need and get reimbursed for it?

It is important to learn about the various types of health insurance available and the benefits they offer. The most common type of health insurer is the indemnity insurer. This type of insurance company typically reimburses you for the portion of the medical bill above and beyond your copayment. When you start a new job, there is the issue of preexisting conditions, which the insurer may not cover for up to twelve months. This can include migraine headaches.

Even when a medical condition is covered, the insurer may reject claims for procedures and tests ordered to rule out other conditions. Claims adjusters usually interpret the rules in the strictest sense, but are willing to listen to a valid appeal. The best way to fight a claim rejection is persistence. Repeated appeals may be the difference between getting the insurance company to pay or being stuck with a prohibitive medical bill. Recent state and federal laws, along with a growing number of successful lawsuits, have forced the health insurance industry to rethink its business practices.

Don't allow your policy to lapse. Insurance companies can't drop you because you develop a new medical problem, but you can be dropped if your policy lapses. It can prove very difficult to get new health insurance after you've been diagnosed with a chronic problem.

If you plan to change jobs, do your research. If you can't take your insurance to your new job, check to make sure your new job will cover your preexisting condition. In some cases, if you have to leave your job, you may be entitled to continued coverage if you pay the premium and an administrative fee. If you are unemployed and don't have health insurance, check with your state's insurance commission for help.

Dealing with Managed-Care Networks, Medicare, and Medicaid

Most insured Americans get their health care from health maintenance organizations (HMOs), preferred provider organizations (PPOs), and independent practice associations (IPAs). These managed-care providers aim to provide quality, comprehensive health care at the lowest possible cost. Their plans use primary care physicians and other providers as "gatekeepers," referring patients to medical and surgical specialists only when absolutely necessary.

Criticisms leveled at managed-care organizations have to do with the quality and volume of care available to patients with complicated health problems. Many patients afflicted with complicated illnesses—such as recalcitrant migraine headaches—charge that HMOs and other managed-care providers make it difficult for them to obtain timely care from specialists.

As stated earlier, persistence and repeated appeals may be the difference between settling for a less-than-appealing doctor-patient relationship and getting a better deal within your managed-care organization. A number of successful lawsuits have forced an industry-wide review of business practices. Managed-care bureaucrats are now willing to listen to members who press their cases for reviews and hearings.

Like managed-care providers and health insurance companies, government-sponsored Medicare and Medicaid insurance coverage can prove to be very frustrating. Medicare is a federally funded program that pays part of the health care cost for individuals aged sixty-five years and older, and people with a disability that qualifies them for Social Security Disability Insurance (SSDI).

Medicaid is a combination local, state, and federally funded insurance program that covers people with income levels below the poverty line. People who qualify for SSDI and Aid to Families with Dependent Children are also eligible for Medicaid.

50. Learn How to Reduce Medication Costs

Taking even a single drug every day for the rest of your life can prove costly, and it really becomes cost prohibitive if you take multiple medications daily. Selling drugs is big business for pharmaceutical companies. The over-the-counter painkiller market alone is worth $2.7 billion annually. If you're being prescribed medications for the first time, ask your doctor for samples. This allows you time before investing your money to get your dosage adjusted, and to see if you respond to this particular drug or develop adverse reactions to it. Sometimes the medication you are originally prescribed is not the one you stay on in the long run.

When you are given a new prescription, ask your practitioner to allow refills on the prescription. Refills will save you the added expense of additional doctor visits just to get a prescription written. Using coupons can also help you save with each purchase. Ask your doctor, nurse, or pharmacist for the coupons they frequently get from drug salespersons. Your pharmacist can also provide you with the address of the company that manufactures your drug, and you can write to its sales/public relations department for discount coupons.

Buying in Bulk

There are now many reputable mail-order drug distributors that sell medications at reduced prices, sometimes 10 to 35 percent cheaper than local pharmacies. The biggest advantages of buying in bulk are the convenience of mail-order shopping and the availability of a list of prices for comparison.

One drawback of buying in bulk is the risk of your drug expiring before you are able to finish using it. To prevent this, buy only a three-month or six-month supply, and always check the expiration date on your medication when it arrives. Most mail-order drug companies will exchange pills if you anticipate they will expire before you can use them.

How About Generic Drugs?

Upon expiration of a drug company's patent on a drug (usually after seventeen years), other companies are free to make the drug from its patent chemical components. Per regulations, generic drug manufacturers are required to ensure that their drug product is adequately absorbed and distributed in the body, but they are not required to conduct rigorous testing to see if the generic version is comparable to the original agent. The question remains whether the generic form of the drug is as potent as the brand-name form. This is an issue that has been hotly debated for some time now and one you should bring up with your doctor.

Generic drugs are usually cheaper than the brand-name form of the same drug. If your physician feels that the generic form of the agent you are prescribed is comparable to the brand-name form, you may want to buy generic and save some money. The proof will be in the pudding; if your headaches return after switching to a generic, then you'll want to stick to the brand-name drug.

If you switch to a generic, remember that it is possible that the generic may cause new drug-associated symptoms such as heartburn or constipation. If this occurs, bring your concern to the attention of your doctor. Conversely, the generic may have fewer side effects. It is also likely that the pill will be a different color and shape from your brand-name drug. The color and shape of a drug has nothing to do with its efficacy. Each drug manufacturer decides what color and shape to make its pills. Manufacturers choose color and shape based on the thinking that a certain color (e.g., red) and shape (e.g., a football shape) may enhance the pill's psychological potency.

Conclusion

Developing a Comprehensive Plan

If you haven't already done so, write down a plan of action. Starting with the types of headaches you get, your plan should include when they occur; why they occur; which foods trigger an attack; which drug, herbal, or nondrug therapy works best for you; and when to consult your health care provider. The following is a recommended comprehensive plan to control your migraines.

- Learn all you can about migraines in general and your specific headaches in particular.

- Find a good health care professional versed in taking care of migraines. A good clinician is willing to educate the patient about his or her condition.

- Learn how to clearly and completely communicate the extent and impact of your headaches. Using the headache symptom diary in Appendix A will help you to do this.

- Learn what your headache triggers are and avoid them at all cost. Your headache diary will help you to do this.

- Exploit the full limits of nondrug strategies such as the mind/body therapies.

- Take your medication or medicinal herb as prescribed. Do not overuse medications.

- If advisable, educate your friends, relatives, coworkers, and supervisor about your condition.

A Look to the Future

What's next for you as you develop the skills to rid yourself of your migraines? I suggest a stepwise implementation of the strategies that best suit you. Please remember that it takes time to conquer long-standing medical problems such as migraines. If you've suffered with migraines for ten years, it'll take more than a few days to get rid of them. Be patient, ask all the right questions of your health care team, seek your providers' advice, read this book as many times as it takes, and stick with your plan.

Scientists and clinicians are constantly seeking clues to the migraine puzzle, pharmaceutical companies continue to develop new migraine drugs, and herbalists are working hard to find effective medicinal herbs with which to manage migraine headaches. Because scientific research and clinical observation are predicted to provide new insight and improved ways of managing old problems, I expect that some information in this book will soon become obsolete. I'll stay abreast of these changes and will include them in future editions of *50 Ways to Control Migraines.* You should also keep abreast of current headache information and watch for developments announced by print and television media, as well as information found on the Internet. Be sure to keep your doctor informed of any and all treatments you plan to implement.

Appendix A

Headache Symptom Diary

Your headache symptom diary helps you detail your headache pain and associated symptoms. It need not be elaborate, but accuracy is important. Write down all your observations for about four to six weeks. The importance of your symptoms may not be evident at the time they occur, but after you have recorded everything, the pattern and timing of your symptoms may tell a compelling story. In addition to helping your doctor to diagnose the type of headache you might have, it will also help him or her plan a treatment strategy that's right for you.

Name: _____ Date: _____

Current medications: _____

Allergies/sensitivities: _____

1. Drugs _____

2. Seasonal _____

3. Food _____

How many cups of coffee/tea/cola beverages do you
consume per day? _____

Do you smoke? If so, how many packs per day? _____

How many alcoholic beverages do you drink per week? _____

Time headache began: _____ Time headache ended: _____

Weather conditions: _____

_____

Warning signs or symptoms (e.g., seeing flashing lights or blind
spots): _____

_____

_____

Associated signs or symptoms (e.g., nausea, vomiting, diarrhea):

_____

_____

First day of menstrual period: _____

Intensity of pain: (mild) 1 2 3 4 5 6 7 8 9 10 (severe)

Location of headache: _____

_____

Foods and drinks consumed today and time consumed:

_____

_____

Activities and time of day: _____

_____

Miscellaneous observations: _____

_____

Self-treatments and their effects: _____

_____

Appendix B

Migraine Headache Resources

An important aspect of being a proactive partner in the management of any chronic disease is knowing where to find additional information. Many consumer, governmental, and health organizations offer valuable information about migraine headache at little or no cost to consumers. Feel free to contact these organizations by writing to them or via telephone or Internet access.

Headache Information

American Council for Headache Education (ACHE)
875 Kings Highway, Suite 200
Woodbury, NJ 08096
1-800-255-ACHE
www.achenet.org

The ACHE is a nonprofit support organization for headache sufferers and their families. It dedicates its resources to educating the public, health care professionals, insurance companies, and legislators about headache, and supports research into all forms of headaches.

National Headache Foundation
423 West St. James Place, 2nd Floor
Chicago, IL 60614-2750
1-800-843-2256; in Illinois, 1-800-523-8858
www.headaches.org

M.A.G.N.U.M., Inc.
(Migraine Awareness Group: A National Understanding for Migraineurs)
113 South Saint Asaph, Suite 300
Alexandria, VA 22314
(703) 739-9384; fax: (703) 739-2432
www.migraines.org

American Chronic Pain Association
P.O. Box 850
Rocklin, CA 95677-0850
(916) 632-3208
www.theacpa.org

American Medical Association (AMA)
515 North State Street
Chicago, IL 60610
(312) 464-4804; fax: (312) 464-4184
www.ama-asn.org/special/migraine

The largest physician advocate organization in the United States, the AMA maintains a comprehensive clearinghouse on a wide range of health topics, including recurrent headaches.

American Osteopathic Association
142 East Ontario Street
Chicago, IL 60611
1-800-621-1773
www.aoa-net.org

American Academy of Pediatrics
141 Northwest Point Boulevard
Elk Grove, IL 60007-1098
(847) 434-4000
www.aap.org

The largest organization representing the interests of American pediatricians, the AAP maintains an extensive catalog of diseases affecting children, including headaches.

American Chiropractic Association
1701 Clarendon Boulevard
Arlington, VA 22201
1-800-986-4636
www.amerchiro.org

The largest organization representing the interests of American chiropractors, the ACA provides information on diseases that are amenable to chiropractic care, and facilitates referrals to chiropractors.

American Physical Therapy Association
1111 North Fairfax Street
Alexandria, VA 22314
(703) 684-2782
www.goldengate-cpta.org

Migraine Association of Canada
>365 Bloor Street, Suite 1912
>Toronto, ON M4W 3L4
>(416) 920-4916 or 1-800-663-3557
>24-hour information line: (416) 920-4917
>fax: (416) 920-3677
>E-mail: support@migraine.can

Drug Information

Food and Drug Administration (FDA)
>HFD-8
>Rockville, MD 20857
>(301) 295-8012

The FDA regulates the research, manufacture, sale, and consumption of all drugs in the United States.

Nonprescription Drug Manufacturers Association (NDMA)
>1150 Connecticut Avenue, NW
>Washington, DC 20036

A national organization representing companies dedicated to providing consumers with over-the-counter (OTC) medications. The NDMA is also an excellent resource for information about the indication, contraindication, efficacy, safety, and adverse effects of OTCs.

Nutrition Information

American Dietetic Association
216 West Jackson Boulevard
Chicago, IL 60606
1-800-877-1600
www.eatright.org

This organization provides information about nutrition and can also help you find a registered dietitian in your area.

Complementary and Alternative Medicine Information

National Center for Complementary and Alternative Medicine (NCCAM)
P.O. Box 8218
Silver Spring, MD 20907-8218
1-888-644-6226
www.nccam.nih.gov

The NCCAM is a U.S. government agency established by Congress in 1998 to stimulate, develop, and support research on CAM for the benefit of the public. The NCCAM advocates for quality science, and rigorous and relevant research into CAM therapies.

American Association of Naturopathic Physicians
8201 Greensboro Drive, Suite 300
McLean, VA 22102
(703) 610-9037
www.naturopathic.org

This organization represents licensed naturopathic physicians (N.D.s) in the United States. Its members are graduates of one of the three American naturopathic medical schools.

American Naturopathic Medical Association
P.O. Box 96273
Las Vegas, NV 89193
(702) 897-7053
www.anma.com

This organization advocates for traditional naturopaths (N.D.s) and other practitioners who use naturopathic principles to help the body stay well.

American Institute of Homeopathy
801 North Fairfax, Suite 306
Alexandria, VA 22314
(703) 246-9501

This nonprofit organization, dedicated to the advancement of the practice of homeopathy, provides a directory of pharmacies and practitioners specializing in homeopathic medicine in the United States.

Homeopathic Academy of Naturopathic Physicians
12132 SE Foster Place
Portland, OR 97266
(503) 761-3298
www.healthy.net

National Commission for the Certification of Acupuncturists
1424 16th Street, NW, Suite 601
Washington, DC 20036
(202) 232-1404

This organization certifies acupuncturists via a standard examination. The organization provides information to the public on the practice of acupuncture.

American Association of Oriental Medicine
433 Front Street
Catasauqua, PA 18032
(610) 260-1433
www.aaom.org

American Massage Therapy Association
820 Davis Street
Evanston, IL 60201
(847) 864-0123
www.amtamassage.org

This association advocates for practitioners of therapeutic massage, provides information to the public, and facilitates referrals to massage therapists throughout the United States.

National Certification Board for Therapeutic Massage and Bodywork (NCBTMB)
8201 Greensboro Drive, Suite 300
McLean, VA 22102
1-800-296-0664 or (703) 610-9015
www.ncbtmb.com

International Association of Yoga Therapists
109 Hillside Avenue
Mill Valley, CA 94941
(415) 383-4587

This nonprofit organization, dedicated to the advancement of the practice of yoga, funds research and educates the public about yoga and its many benefits.

International Institute of Reflexology
P.O. Box 12642
St. Petersburg, FL 33733-2642
(813) 343-4811

This institute disseminates general information, books, and pamphlets about reflexology. It also conducts seminars and training on reflexology and makes referrals to reflexology practitioners throughout the United States.

The Institute of Transpersonal Psychology
744 San Antonio Road
Palo Alto, CA 94303
(415) 493-4430

This institute provides information, conducts imagery training, and certifies persons interested in mind/body consciousness.

Center for Mind/Body Medicine
5225 Connecticut Avenue NW, Suite 414
Washington, DC 20015
(202) 966-7338

Notes

Introduction

1. J. Paulino and C. J. Griffith, *The Headache Sourcebook* (Chicago: Contemporary Books, 2001).
2. See note 1.
3. The National Headache Foundation, *Managing Headaches: What You Need to Know* (Chicago: National Headache Foundation, 1999).
4. The American Council for Headache Education, with L. M. Constantine and S. Scott, *Migraine: The Complete Guide* (New York: Dell Publishing Group, Inc., 1994).

Part One

1. A. M. Rapoport and F. D. Sheftell, *Headache Relief* (New York: Fireside, 1991).
2. C. Gorman, "Oh, my aching head!" *Time* (30 June 1997): 62.
3. M. B. Stevens, "Tension-Type Headaches," *American Family Physician* 47 (1993): 799–805.
4. See note 3.
5. Headache Classification Committee of the International Headache Society, "Classification and Diagnostic Criteria

for Headache Disorders, Cranial Neuralgias, and Facial Pain," *Cephalgia* 8 (1988): 1–96.

6. C. B. Inlander and P. Shimer, *Headaches: 47 Ways to Stop the Pain* (New York: St. Martin's Press, 1995).

7. The National Headache Foundation, *Managing Headaches: What You Need to Know* (Chicago: National Headache Foundation, 1999).

8. J. W. Lance, *Headache: Understanding Alleviation* (New York: Charles Scribner's Sons, 1975).

9. G. E. R. Lloyd, ed., *Hippocratic Writings* (London: Penguin Books, Ltd., 1983).

10. E. H. Ackernecht, *A Short History of Medicine* (Baltimore: The Johns Hopkins University Press, 1982).

11. See note 10.

12. A. Elkind, *Migraines: Everything You Need to Know About Their Cause and Cure* (New York: Avon Books, 1983).

13. The American Council for Headache Education, with L. M. Constantine and S. Scott, *Migraine: The Complete Guide* (New York: Dell Publishing Group, Inc., 1994).

14. P. Maas and D. Mitchell, *Guide to Headache Relief* (New York: Pocket Books, 1997).

15. See note 10.

16. G. Selby and J. W. Lance, "Observation of 500 Cases of Migraine and Allied Vascular Headache," *Journal of Neurological and Neurosurgical Psychiatry* 23 (1960).

17. See note 12.

18. C. Peterson, *The Women's Migraine Survival Guide* (New York: HarperCollins, 1999).

19. S. Dyson, *Migraines: A Natural Approach* (Berkeley, CA: Ulysses Press, 1998).

20. See note 13.

21. S. L. Burks, *Managing Your Migraine: A Migraine Sufferer's Practical Guide* (New Jersey: Humana Press, Inc., 1994).

22. S. D. Silberstein and J. Saper, "Migraine: Diagnosis and Treatment," *Wolff's Headache and Other Head Pain* (New York: Oxford University Press, 1993).

23. See note 13.

24. See note 13.
25. F. Fracchinetti et al., "Magnesium Prophylaxis of Menstrual Migraine Effects of Intracellular Magnesium," *Headache* (1991): 298–301.
26. A. Mauskop, *What Your Doctor May Not Tell You About Migraines* (New York: Warner Books, 2001).
27. See note 1.
28. See note 13.
29. See note 13.
30. See note 13.
31. See note 1.
32. See note 13.
33. See note 13.
34. See note 12.
35. See note 13.
36. See note 5.
37. See note 12.
38. R. S. Kunkel, "Managing Primary Headache Syndromes," *Patient Care* (2000): 100–122.
39. S. Diamond and M. A. Franklin, *Conquering Your Migraine* (New York: Fireside Books, 2001).
40. W. J. Stoffey, "Headaches," *PA Today* 6 (1998): 8–13.
41. See note 3.
42. Modified from J. Paulino and C. J. Griffith, *The Headache Sourcebook* (Chicago: Contemporary Books, 2001).

Part Two

1. C. Peterson, *The Women's Migraine Survival Guide* (New York: HarperCollins, 1999).
2. The American Council for Headache Education, with L. M. Constantine and S. Scott, *Migraine: The Complete Guide* (New York: Dell Publishing Group, Inc., 1994).
3. See note 1.
4. P. Maas and D. Mitchell, *Guide to Headache Relief* (New York: Pocket Books, 1997).
5. See note 1.

6. A. M. Rapoport and F. D. Sheftell, *Headache Relief* (New York: Fireside, 1991).
7. See note 6.
8. See note 6.
9. See note 6.
10. See note 6.
11. See note 6.
12. See note 2.
13. See note 2.
14. P. Winner, "Teens Prone to Monday Migraines," *Clinician Review* 10 (2000): 95–103.
15. See note 2.
16. See note 2.

Part Three

1. P. Maas and D. Mitchell, *Guide to Headache Relief* (New York: Pocket Books, 1997).

Part Four

1. J. Paulino and C. J. Griffith, *The Headache Sourcebook* (Chicago: Contemporary Books, 2001).
2. See note 1.
3. P. Maas and D. Mitchell, *Guide to Headache Relief* (New York: Pocket Books, 1997).
4. D. M. Eisenberg et al., "Trends in Alternative Medicine Use in the United States, 1990–1997: Results of a Follow-Up National Survey," *Journal of the American Medical Association* 280 (1998): 1569–75.
5. M. Knaster, *Discovering the Body's Wisdom* (New York: Bantam Books, 1996).
6. The National Headache Foundation, *Managing Headaches: What You Need to Know* (Chicago: National Headache Foundation, 1999).

Part Five

1. S. Wood and B. Griffith, *Conquering High Blood Pressure* (New York: Perseus Books, 1997).
2. See note 1.
3. P. Maas and D. Mitchell, *Guide to Headache Relief* (New York: Pocket Books, 1997).
4. A. M. Rapoport and F. D Sheftell, *Headache Relief for Women* (Boston: Little, Brown and Co., 1995).
5. See note 1.
6. C. C. Tollison and J. W. Tollison, *Headache: A Multimodal Program for Relief* (New York: Sterling Publishing Co., Inc., 1982).
7. See note 4.
8. See note 4.
9. L. Lane, "Nutritionist Calls for Tighter Regulation of Supplements," at www.cnn.comHEALTH/alternative/9909/17/supplement.drug.journal (accessed May 23, 2000).
10. R. B. Ervin, J. D Wright, and J. Kennedy-Stephenson, "Use of Dietary Supplements in the United States: 1988–1994," *Vital Health Statistics* 24 (1999): 1–14.
11. J. Graedon and T. Graedon, *The People's Pharmacy Guide to Home and Herbal Remedies* (New York: St. Martin's Griffin, 2001).
12. See note 10.
13. See note 11.
14. E. Urbaniak, *Natural Healing for Headaches* (Gig Harbor, WA: Harbor Press, 2000).
15. See note 4.

Glossary

Abortive headache drug Medication used to stop (abort) a headache after the head pain has begun.

Acupressure Also known as shiatsu, this is a type of deep massage using the fingertips, palms, elbows, knees, and feet to stimulate the acupuncture points to produce the same results as acupuncture.

Acupuncture An ancient Chinese treatment using hair-thin needles to restore the free flow of bioenergy through channels called meridians.

Adrenaline Also called epinephrine, adrenaline is the "fight or flight" hormone secreted by the adrenal glands, which sit atop the kidneys. It can quickly increase heart rate and blood pressure in response to emotional or physical threat.

Aerobic exercise Physical activity that enhances the body's intake and utilization of oxygen. An important aspect of cardiovascular fitness, aerobic exercise includes jogging, running, swimming, walking, and bicycling.

Amines A group of nitrogen-based proteins implicated as triggers of migraine and other types of vascular headaches.

159

Anaerobic exercise   Exercise whose energy comes from burning fat without the use of oxygen. Examples include isometrics and weight lifting.

Analgesics   A class of medications, commonly known as painkillers, that are used to relieve pain. Examples include aspirin, acetaminophen (e.g., Tylenol), and ibuprofen.

Aneurysm   A bulge in the wall of an artery due to weakening of the wall by disease or birth defect that is at risk of rupturing.

Angiogram   A specialized study of the carotid and other arteries in which dye is injected into the bloodstream and x-rays are taken as the fluid travels through the blood vessels to the head and neck. The dye enhances the structures within the arteries. (See *Arteriogram.*)

Antidepressants   A group of medications developed to treat depression that have been found to be effective at treating migraine headache.

Arteries   Blood vessels that carry blood away from the heart to different parts of the body.

Arteriogram   A diagnostic x-ray of the arteries taken after the injection of contrast dye into the bloodstream to make the blood vessels more visible. (See *Angiogram.*)

Aura   A symptom or set of symptoms, such as flashing lights, zigzag lines, or temporary loss of vision, that can signal the onset of some forms of migraines (called migraine with aura).

Basilar artery migraine   A rare form of migraine, occurring mostly in young women, adolescents, and children, that is caused by disturbance in a major brain artery. Symptoms include loss of balance, difficulty speaking, double vision, poor muscle coordination, and occasionally loss of consciousness.

Beta-blocker A drug that blocks the effects of selective body hormones (e.g., epinephrine) on the heart and blood vessels. These agents slow the heart rate, lower blood pressure, and reduce the heart's oxygen requirements. This last effect makes them ideal for treating patients with angina pectoris. Some of these agents narrow the bronchial (airway) tubes and may exacerbate asthma.

Biofeedback Immediate information about a bodily function (such as heartbeat or muscle tension) through audiovisual feedback that allows a person to change the level of that bodily function through relaxation and other methods of operant conditioning.

Blood pressure The pressure created by the circulating blood on the walls of the arteries. Blood pressure results from the contraction, or squeezing, of the heart vis-à-vis the resistance put up by the circumference of the blood vessels. Many hormones, enzymes, and blood vessel structures influence blood pressure. Blood pressure is also influenced by the volume of circulating blood.

Blood vessels The network of tubes (arteries, veins, and capillaries) that carry blood through the body.

Brain scan A specialized study in which a radioactive chemical (called a radionuclide) is injected in the arm and travels to the brain, enhancing its outline when x-rays are taken.

Caffeine A stimulant substance found in tea, coffee, cola, and other products. Caffeine withdrawal and excessive use can trigger migraines. Caffeine is also an ingredient in some migraine medications.

Calcium channel blocker A blood pressure–lowering drug that works by blocking calcium from entering through microscopic channels in the walls of arteries. This blockade results in relaxation of the arterial walls, thereby lowering blood pressure. This drug is also used to reduce the frequency and severity of migraine headaches.

Carotid arteries   The two main arteries that supply blood to the head and neck.

Cephalgia   The medical term for headache or pain in the head.

Cervicogenic headache   A type of secondary headache caused by arthritis and other conditions of the bones and joints in the neck.

Cholesterol   A waxy substance produced by the body (and also found in animal fat and dairy products) that is necessary for the production of hormones and cell function.

Cluster headache   A type of vascular headache so named because of its repeated occurrences in groups or clusters. These severely painful headaches, most common among men, are typically located around one eye and are associated with tearing and a runny nose.

Computerized axial tomography (CAT) scan   An x-ray procedure that produces a computer-enhanced picture of a cross section of the body, creating three-dimensional images of internal organs and body structures.

Constriction   Narrowing of blood vessels caused by contraction of their muscles.

Coronary artery disease   Disease affecting the arteries that supply blood to the heart muscle. The most common type of coronary artery disease is atherosclerosis—the deposit of fat, cholesterol, and calcium on the inner walls of the coronary arteries.

Corticosteroids   Steroid hormones secreted by the adrenal glands that help to prevent or reduce inflammation. These drugs are used to prevent and treat vascular headaches.

Dihydroergotamine   A drug used to treat migraine and cluster headaches.

Electroencephalography   Also referred to as an EEG, this test delineates the electrical activity of nerve cells in the brain via electrodes applied to the scalp. An EEG can provide information regarding disorders of the brain such as seizures, tumors, and blood clots.

Electronystagmography   Also referred to as an ENG, this test records eye movements by measuring the electrical impulses of the eye muscles. Generally, ENGs are used to detect tumors on the nerves that serve the eye muscles.

Endocrine system   A system of glands that manufacture hormones. Endocrine glands include the thyroid gland, the adrenal glands, the ovaries, and the testes.

Endorphins   Morphinelike chemicals naturally secreted by the nervous system. These amino-acid–based chemicals are abundantly produced during aerobic exercise and have an important role in pain reduction.

Epinephrine   Also called adrenaline, this hormone has important functions in the regulation of blood pressure. (See *Adrenaline.*)

Ergotamine tartrate   A drug used to treat migraine headaches.

Estrogen   One of the female sex hormones that is produced primarily by the ovaries during a woman's childbearing years. Estrogen prepares the wall of the uterus for implantation of the fertilized egg. Estrogen is used in birth control pills to prevent pregnancy and in hormone replacement pills to treat the effects of menopause.

Heart rate   Reflected by the pulse, the heart rate refers to the number of times the heart pumps blood per minute.

High blood pressure   See *Hypertension.*

Hormones   Substances secreted by an endocrine gland that influence the activities of various organs (e.g., estrogen secreted by the ovaries helps give a woman her feminizing features).

Hormone replacement therapy   Hormones taken by women after a hysterectomy or menopause to prevent osteoporosis (bone thinning) and heart disease.

Hypertension   Abnormally high blood pressure within the blood vessels caused by increased volume of circulating blood and/or decreased diameter of the blood vessels, among other factors. Hypertension and high blood pressure are interchangeable terms.

Hyperthyroidism   Abnormally high production of thyroid hormone by the thyroid gland that sits at the base of the front of the neck.

Hypotension   Low blood pressure, defined as blood pressure below 100/60.

Ice cream headache   A type of headache caused by cooling of the tissues in the roof of the mouth by eating ice cream or other cold substances.

Internists   Physicians who have at least three years of training beyond medical school. These doctors restrict their practice to matters of internal medicine, which includes conditions such as high blood pressure, diabetes, and headache. Do not confuse these practitioners with interns, who are newly graduated physicians-in-training.

Isometric exercise   Exercise that involves applying bodily force against stable resistance (e.g., weight lifting).

Low blood pressure   See *Hypotension*.

Lumbar puncture   Commonly referred to as a spinal tap, this diagnostic test involves removing a small amount of spinal fluid using a needle inserted in the spinal canal in the lower back. Spinal taps are used to help diagnose conditions such as meningitis, brain hemorrhage, and other life-threatening conditions.

Magnesium   A metallic element that is crucial to the function of bones, muscles, nerves, and other bodily tissues.

Magnetic resonance imaging (MRI) scan   A highly specialized imaging technique that uses magnets and computers to form a three-dimensional image of internal organs, such as the brain.

Meningitis   An infection of the membranes covering the brain and spinal cord.

Menstrual migraine   A migraine attack that occurs during the menstrual cycle.

Migraine headache   A type of neurovascular headache caused by biochemical changes and inflammation in the brain and associated blood vessels that lead to the widening and narrowing of blood vessels that feed the head and neck.

Migraineur   A person who suffers from migraine headaches.

Monoamine oxidase   A family of enzymes that are involved in the breakdown of neurotransmitters.

Monoamine-oxidase (MAO) inhibitors   A group of antidepressant drugs that increase the body's level of mood-elevating chemicals (such as norepinephrine) by preventing their breakdown. People taking MAO inhibitors should refrain from consuming foods or drinks containing tyramine, such as red wine, aged cheese, and overripe bananas.

Monosodium glutamate (MSG)   A food flavor enhancer commonly found in packaged and canned goods and frozen entrées sold in supermarkets.

Musculoskeletal   Having to do with the bones, muscles, ligaments, tendons, and other components of the body's skeletal system.

Nephropathy   A reduction in the kidneys' ability to clear the body of waste products due to damage from a number of factors including certain drugs, diabetes mellitus, and other diseases.

Neurotransmitters   The chemical messengers—e.g., serotonin, dopamine, and norepinephrine—that facilitate communication between brain cells.

Neurovascular   Having to do with both the nerves (*neuro*) and blood vessels (*vascular*).

Nicotine   A stimulant substance contained in cigarettes and other tobacco products. Nicotine can trigger migraine headaches by narrowing blood vessels that go to the head and neck.

Nitrates   A group of chemicals used to preserve meat and prevent food from spoiling and as preservatives in many canned foods. Also referred to as nitrites.

Nitrites   See *Nitrates*.

Nonsteroidal anti-inflammatory drugs (NSAIDs)   Drugs used to treat the pain and inflammation associated with headaches such as ibuprofen and naproxen.

Nurse practitioner   A nurse with advanced training to perform many health care tasks traditionally provided by a physician.

Ophthalmoplegic migraine   A rare form of migraine that causes double vision and the eyelid to droop.

Pain threshold   The weakest stimulus at which a sensation is felt and interpreted by an individual as pain.

Pain tolerance   The degree of severity each person assigns a pain stimulus.

Positron emission tomogram (PET) scan A computer-enhanced study that uses radioactive particles (called positrons) to study the function of the brain. A sugar solution containing a radioactive "tag" is swallowed and carried to the brain. X-rays are then taken of the areas tagged with positrons to look for brain tumors, blood clots, and other conditions.

Physician assistant (PA) A health care professional who, by formal training and experience, performs many medical functions traditionally performed by physicians. Studies have shown that primary care PAs can effectively carry out between 80 percent and 90 percent of the tasks performed by general-practice physicians.

Pituitary gland A pea-sized gland that sits at the base of the skull. It secretes numerous hormones, including vasopressin and others that regulate blood pressure.

Placebo An inactive substance given under the pretext of a real drug.

Plaque Fatty deposits in the blood vessels that reduce the free flow of blood.

Potassium A vital electrolyte found in the blood and cells that plays a key role in the function of nerves and muscles, including the heart muscle. Potassium can be found in foods such as orange juice and bananas.

Prednisone An artificial cortisone drug used to prevent and treat vascular headaches. (See *Corticosteroids*.)

Prognosis A prediction regarding the expected course of a disease process.

Pseudotumor cerebri A condition in which there is abnormally high pressure in the spinal fluid that bathes the brain and spinal cord. The exact cause of pseudotumor cerebri is unknown, but the condition is associated with certain other conditions (such as pregnancy and head injury), vitamin A deficiency, and the use of certain medications (such as tetracycline, sulfonamides, and indomethacin).

Reflexology A form of massage therapy that applies pressure to the feet, palms, and ears to cause relaxation. Practitioners of this therapy claim to help treat chronic constipation, asthma, and chronic headaches, among other conditions.

Risk factor A condition and or habit that incurs increased likelihood of developing a disease. Obesity, smoking, high alcohol intake, and excessive sodium consumption are among the most prevalent risk factors for high blood pressure.

Selective serotonin reuptake inhibitors (SSRIs) A class of antidepressants that selectively concentrate on the part of the brain influenced by serotonin. SSRIs have fewer side effects than older antidepressants, such as the MAO inhibitors.

Serotonin A neurotransmitter found in the brain that transmits information about blood flow in the brain and pain chemicals found in brain fluids.

Sinusitis Inflammation of the sinus cavities located around the eyes and nostrils.

Sleep apnea Transient stoppage of breathing while asleep. Its causes include obesity, and it can lead to high blood pressure.

Sodium A mineral element that, in the body, controls water balance, nerve impulse, muscle contraction, and acid-base balance. Approximately 40 percent of table salt (chemical name, sodium chloride) is sodium. People who are salt sensitive run the risk of developing high blood pressure if they consume large quantities of sodium.

Spinal tap See *Lumbar puncture*.

Steroids See *Corticosteroids*.

Stress The response to perceived threat to our psychological or physical well-being, and the realization that we lack the resources necessary to cope with that threat.

Stroke Also referred to as cerebrovascular accident, or CVA. Stroke is a sudden loss of function of a part of the brain due to cessation of blood flow caused by a blood vessel rupture (hemorrhage) or blockage (a clot). Strokes can lead to paralysis and death. Hypertension is the most important risk factor for stroke.

Symptom A pain, weakness, or something felt or noticed by the patient that indicates that a disease or disorder is affecting the body.

Temporal arteritis A condition caused by the thickening of the walls of the arteries that feed the temples and eyes. Its cause is unknown and it produces headaches, scalp sensitivity, and altered vision. It is associated with a condition called polymyalgia rheumatica.

Temporomandibular joint (TMJ) dysfunction An inflammation of the joint between the temporal bone and lower jaw (located just in front of the ear) that can cause headaches. Symptoms include pain, and clicking and locking of the jaw.

Transcutaneous electrical nerve stimulation (TENS) A treatment modality that uses electrical signals to stimulate nerve endings to control pain.

Tricyclic antidepressants A group of antidepressants that elevate mood by manipulating the body's level of the mood-elevating chemical norepinephrine.

Trigeminal neuralgia A painful condition of the trigeminal nerve. Symptoms include intense facial pain. Also referred to as tic douloureux.

Triggers Factors that set off a condition. In the case of cluster headaches, alcohol and nicotine are common triggers. Some migraine headaches are triggered by noise and flickering lights.

Tumor   A growth or enlargement of a tissue that can be cancerous or benign (harmless).

Tyramine   A nitrogen-based protein component found in aged foods such as cheese, yogurt, buttermilk, and overripe bananas, and implicated as a migraine headache trigger.

Vascular   Refers to blood vessels (arteries, veins, arterioles, and capillaries) that carry blood throughout the body.

Vascular headaches   Headaches caused by abnormal functioning of the body's blood vessels. Migraine and cluster headaches are considered vascular headaches.

Vasoactive   Refers to the ability to cause the widening or narrowing of blood vessels. Caffeine, nicotine, and adrenaline are vasoactive substances, as are medications such as nitroglycerine, hydralazine, and nitroprusside.

Vasodilators   Drugs that dilate, or increase, the circumference of the arteries and veins in the body, resulting in a lowering of blood vessel resistance and a reduction in blood pressure.

Veins   Blood vessels that carry blood from the body back to the heart for oxygen replenishment.

Vertigo   A sensation of spinning of one's self or surroundings. It can be caused by a number of conditions, including inner ear inflammation and elevated blood pressure.

Bibliography

Cummings, S., and D. Ullman. *Everybody's Guide to Homeopathic Medicines.* New York: Penguin Putnam, Inc., 1997.

Diamond, S., and M. A. Franklin. *Conquering Your Migraine.* New York: Fireside Books, 2001.

Elkind, A. *Migraines: Everything You Need to Know About Their Cause and Cure.* New York: Avon Books, 1997.

Graedon, J., and T. Graedon. *The People's Pharmacy Guide to Home and Herbal Remedies.* New York: St. Martin's Griffin, 2001.

Hass, E. *The Detox Diet.* Berkeley, CA: Celestial Arts, 1996.

Ingham, E. *Stories the Feet Can Tell thru Reflexology.* Saint Petersburg, FL: Ingham Publishing, Inc., 1984.

Jarney, C., and J. Tindall. *Acupressure for Common Ailments.* New York: Fireside Books, 1991.

Lindlahr, H., and J. Proby, eds. *Philosophy of Natural Therapeutics.* Great Britain: C. W. Daniel Company Limited, 2000.

Mauskop, A., and B. Fox. *What Your Doctor May Not Tell You About Migraines*. New York: Warner Books, 2001.

Paulino, J., and C. J. Griffith. *The Headache Sourcebook*. Chicago: Contemporary Books, 2001.

Peterson, C. *The Women's Migraine Survival Guide*. New York: HarperCollins, 1999.

Rapoport, A. M., and F. D. Sheftell. *Headache Relief for Women*. Boston: Little Brown, 1996.

Roter, D. L., and J. A. Hall. *Doctors Talking with Patients, Patients Talking with Doctors: Improving Communication in Medical Visits*. Westport, CT: Greenwood Publishing Group, 1992.

Stone, U. *Homeopathy for Headaches: Stop Headache Pain the Natural Way*. New York: Kensington Health, 1999.

Swanson, D. *Mayo Clinic on Chronic Pain*. New York: Kensington Publishing Corporation, 1999.

Tappan, F., and P. J. Benjamin. *Tappan's Handbook of Healing Massage Techniques*. Stamford, CT: Appleton & Lange, 1998.

Urbaniak, E. *Natural Healing for Headaches*. Gig Harbor, WA: Harbor Press, 2000.

Index